THE 1918 SPANISH INFLUENZA PANDEMIC

A comprehensive history of the deadliest and most devastating pandemic in human history

A story that teaches us about our past, present, and future

DAVID ANVERSA

I hope you will like this book! If you like, leave a
positive review with your impressions on the Amazon
page.
I would be really grateful! Check my other books in the
Author Page on Amazon, you will find them very
interesting!

For any kind of request, clarification or advice, feel
completely free to contact me at the following email
address: davidanversa.author@gmail.com
Thank you very much and happy reading

David Anversa

Contents:

Understanding Epidemics, Pandemics, and Other Related Terms

When studying epidemiology, which is the study of the incidence, distribution, and control of diseases, we come across a number of terms that help us understand a disease and its magnitude. An epidemic is the outbreak of a disease that affects a multitude of people within a community. The word "epidemic "originates from Greece and it translates to "upon the people." A pandemic is an epidemic that has spread beyond the boundaries of the country of origin to several countries or continents.

Using the ongoing coronavirus pandemic as our example, we understand that when it broke out in Wuhan and was still within China's boundaries, it was still an epidemic. However, when it spread beyond the country's boundaries and spread to other parts of the world, it became a pandemic.

Epidemics are relatively simpler to manage as compared to pandemics given that epidemics affect a relatively smaller group of people over a smaller area. Some diseases are endemic to specific communities, which means that a particular disease is permanent in a specific population. For instance, in the areas surrounding Lake Victoria in Kenya, malaria is endemic to the communities. People in this region have the Sickle-Cell trait, which is an adaptation to resist Plasmodium spp, the pathogen that causes malaria.

Before the coronavirus pandemic, the world has

experienced several pandemics from which we learn lessons concerning the management of diseases and ill health. We see and learn from the mistakes of older generations, and benefit from the advancements of knowledge in medicine, which came to us as a blessing in disguise. We also learn that each disease that afflicts members of society affects almost all aspects of life because health is the total well-being of a person. Disruption of one aspect of health, be it physical, mental, or even spiritual, affects the others. To understand the effects of any pandemic, we have to understand how it affects the afflicted person and the people around this person, the community, the country, and, eventually, the world.

Introduction to the Spanish Flu

Before the 2020 coronavirus pandemic, most of the world's population had no knowledge of the Spanish flu pandemic. The Spanish flu pandemic occurred in 1918 and wreaked havoc on the face of the earth for two years. The origin of the disease has not been well-established to this day. However, France, China, and Britain were among the first countries to report the flu. In the US, the first cases of the disease were reported from a military base in Kansas. One may wonder why the disease is called the Spanish flu as it clearly did not originate from Spain. The reason behind the name is that Spain was a neutral country during the First World War and, therefore, the Spanish government did not censor its media. The state reported all the horrid and terrifying effects of the disease, beginning in late spring of 1918 when a Spanish news service wrote to Reuters in London that a strange form of sickness had appeared in Madrid. This statement created the impression that the disease was specific to the Spanish people, hence the name. Spain lost her leader, King Alfonso, who was among the first people to suffer from this contagion in Spain.

In Spain, the people believed that this malady was brought to them by the French, so hey called it the "French Flu." The disease also has been referred to as the "forgotten pandemic" because the First World War overshadowed its effects. Yet, the Spanish flu pandemic is arguably the most catastrophic misfortune to ever tread the earth. It claimed up to 100 million lives, a far higher amount than the lives lost during both World Wars and the Korean War combined.

The Spanish flu is therefore a significant landmark in history. It altered the social, economic, and political lives of people throughout the world. The effects of the disease were felt even in the most remote areas of the globe.

The Spanish flu was caused by an influenza virus of avian origin. Further research and genome sequencing revealed that the virus was of subtype H1N1. By 1918, viruses had already been discovered by Dmitri Ivanovsky, who is considered to be the father of virology. This basic knowledge of viruses gave people a good starting point in dealing with the Spanish flu. Unlike during previous pandemics when people attributed sickness to the supernatural, people in 1918 were aware of microbes and their effects on the human body. Unfortunately, despite having knowledge of viruses, the causative agent of the Spanish flu was initially mistaken to be a bacteria named Pfeiffer's bacillus. The German bacteriologist Richard Pfeiffer had isolated the bacillus in people who suffered from severe influenza. He named the bacillus Haemophilus influenzae. This bacillus had caused the Russian flu, which occurred before the Spanish flu. This bacteria was also isolated in some of the patients who contracted the Spanish flu. On September 28th, 1918, some Spanish newspapers attempted to educate the masses concerning the disease, its causative agent, and how to remain safe. Despite all these efforts, the scourge afflicted people with such viciousness that they found themselves utterly helpless. It was only in 1933 that scientists were able to identify and isolate the virus that causes influenza in human beings.

They also discovered that Pfeiffer's bacillus causes many infections such as pneumonia and meningitis, but not influenza.

The first recorded case of the Spanish flu was at the Camp Funston military base in Kansas. It is believed that as the soldiers sailed to Europe in their unsanitary and crowded ships, the disease spread to other soldiers and occupants of the vessels. Upon reaching Europe, the virus had already been incubated and was ready to inflict and afflict all people, from the cooks and guards at the camp, the soldiers on the battlefield, and civilians.

The disease spread to German, French, British, and other military bases that were participating in the World War. Eventually, it made its way to civilians in both urban and areas.

Some called the Spanish flu the Sandfly Fever while others called it the Purple Death. All in all, the disease had characteristic signs and symptoms. Similar to the common cold, Spanish Flu manifested in a sore throat, headaches, fevers, and chills. It was also characterized by general fatigue. These symptoms could trick anyone into believing that it was just a common cold and would go away with time. However, as time passed, the symptoms became more severe, and some patients were reported to die only a few hours after contracting the disease. If the patient survived the first few hours, a dry hacking cough would develop that worsened with time. The cough would typically be accompanied by excruciating stomach problems, which consequently led to loss of appetite.

If the ailing person was lucky enough to see a second day after contracting the sickness, they would sweat excessively and likely contract pneumonia or develop other respiratory complications that eventually lead to their death.

This information about the Spanish flu, in a nutshell, will help us understand the propagation of the disease and the overall response to the scourge.

Progress and Propagation of the Spanish Flu

For decades, scientists had been trying to pinpoint the origin of the 1918 Spanish flu pandemic. They had initially concluded that the disease must have originated from France, the US, or Britain. However, according to research carried out by National Geographic, there has been genetic evidence that the disease could have originated in China. Therefore, the question is now, if the Spanish flu originated in China, why were Europe and the US the first regions to be walloped by the pandemic as opposed to Asia?

In 1917, there was a flu-like malady that inflicted people in northern China. Genetic evidence shows that the pathogen causing this strange disease is an ancestral influenza virus. Let us try to understand how virus this could reach other parts of the world, especially the Western world.

During the First World War, China declared itself to be neutral. However, Germany had occupied some parts of China, such as Tsingtao, the most outstanding German overseas naval base. Japan, China's rival since time immemorial, attacked Tsingtao. By doing so, Japan violated China's neutrality and China now had to participate in the war.

For China, choosing which side to join in the war was somewhat mind-racking.

China was fighting primarily against Germany and Japan, who were already rivals, with Germany part of the Central powers and Japan part of the Allies.

Eventually, China sent troops of up to 50,000 people to fight in Europe on the Allies' side. These troops mainly consisted of laborers. The laborers were known as "carrier corps" and they dug trenches to facilitate the movement of soldiers. The Chinese comprised the largest group of non-European troops on the battlefields.

In 1918, as Chinese troops were in Canada en route to Europe, they started coming down with a flu-like disease. However, the physicians dismissed them, claiming that it was an excuse to be exempted from work and even labeling the malady "Chinese laziness." Eventually, most of the Chinese troops ended up in medical quarantine camps rather than in the trenches or on the battlefield. Those who made it to the war fronts were carriers of the flu and transmitted it to the soldiers.

Though the origin of the Spanish flu remains disputable, the course of the disease is well-known and its effects were resoundingly chilling. This scourge did not spare even the remotest areas. Unbeknownst to people at the time, the disease also affected swine, guinea fowls, and other livestock, meaning that people could transmit the flu to animals, who in turn could spread it to other animals and people alike.

The death toll and the misery caused by the pandemic

are hard to fathom. The Spanish flu claimed close to a third of the world's population. However, this figure is said to be much lower than the actual number of people who died due to pandemic.

The Spanish flu occurred in three waves. The first wave of the Spanish flu occurred in spring of 1918, with the initially reported cases coming from Camp Funston in Kansas. The camp's cook, Albert Gitchell, reported to the infirmary complaining of a terrible cold on the morning of March 11th, 1918. This event signaled the start of the first wave of the pandemic. A corporal named Lee Drake also reported to the same infirmary with the same complaint as Gitchell.

By the end of that same day, over a hundred people in the camp had come down with the Spanish flu. In the next few days, other military camps such as Camp Hancock, Camp Sherman, Camp Fremont, and several others reported the same malady.

Despite its mounting cases, the US sent troops of up to 84,000 soldiers, called the "doughboys", to fight against the Germans that March. In May 1918, 118,000 more soldiers were sent to carry out the same task. They were oblivious to the fact that they were the carriers of a virus that was far deadlier than all their missiles. The virus started displaying its viciousness even before the soldiers arrived in Europe. The US had already lost a good number of soldiers by the time the ships carrying the soldiers anchored in Europe.

But in the next few months, the virus gained footholds in both the US and Europe.

Upon the arrival of American troops in Europe, all hell broke loose. The contagion spread like wildfire. It spread far and wide in Europe, all the way to Poland. It affected both sides of the war indiscriminately and caused a change of plans. Besides the US and Europe, the pandemic also impacted virtually every part of the globe, spreading to Africa, India, and Russia, among others. The only regions that did not experience the first wave of the pandemic were Australia and South America.

The first wave of the Spanish flu pandemic is referred to as the "herald wave" because it announced the arrival of the two subsequent waves. This first wave coincided with the general flu season, and, for this reason, most people did not take precautions. However, the media in Spain was not censored since Spain was neutral during the war. Therefore, in the first week of May, Spain reported a strange flu-like malady that had affected many people in Madrid. The spread of the virus in Spain was highly catalyzed by the San Isidro celebrations that were taking place in Madrid. The contagion multiplied rapidly and spread to unsuspecting masses of people. It eventually spread to other parts of the country and affected all people. The San Isidro celebrations unknowingly created the perfect foundation for the spread of the Spanish flu.

Unfortunately, in military camps, the conditions were cramped and unsanitary.

The disease quickly spread from one person to the next. The Spanish flu ended up claiming more soldiers' lives than the First World War itself. The mass troop movements throughout the globe also contributed to the rapid spread of the Spanish flu's first wave. In South Africa, for instance, laborers were reported to go down with an illness that prevented them from working. Soon enough, a third of the laborers were unable to work, and needless to say, this significantly lowered the farms' productivity.

The first wave of the Spanish flu was generally mild and was confused with a bad cold. Patients experienced fever and chills, and many also had a cough, sore throat, and a runny nose. The flu also caused headaches and muscle aches. Some patients complained of fatigue and general malaise. Other patients, especially children, would vomit and experience diarrhea. The Spanish flu's first wave was markedly hard on young children and the elderly. People with preexisting conditions were also at a significant risk of dying due to this disease. However, most young adults in their prime were able to combat the flu and survive it.

The first wave of the Spanish flu had a mortality rate of 0.65 per 1000 people. This wave of the Spanish flu is considered mild because the death rate was almost the same as that of the typical flu season rate in that period. To have a clear picture of this rate, it's helpful to know that in 1915, 65,000 people had died of the flu. Comparatively, during the first wave of the pandemic, only 75,000 people died from the Spanish flu.

Due to this similarity, the actual numbers of those who contracted the Spanish flu in its first wave remain somewhat a mystery. What is known is that the majority of young people acquired, combatted, and defeated the first wave of the Spanish flu due to their more robust immune systems. The effects of the malady were more evident in young children and the elderly.

However, in fall of 1918, the virus came back with a vengeance in its second wave. Scientists suggest that the virus that had caused the first wave of the pandemic had undergone a mutation. The changes that occurred in the virus's structure gave it an upper hand in attacking the human body. Specifically, the virus developed better structures to invade the human body and better mechanisms to evade the actions of the immune system. These changes made the second wave far deadlier than the first wave.

It has been speculated that the second wave of the Spanish flu started in Britain at Port Plymouth. A number of military ships departed from Port Plymouth to other parts of Europe and Africa. These soldiers aboard the ships were not aware that they were carriers of the deadly contagion. In this manner, the virus spread to France, Belgium, Spain, and Liberia, among other countries. Other theories speculate that soldiers who had been carrying out war activities came back home, bringing with them the deadly virus. Other theories conjecture that the Portuguese soldiers who came back from the war had the virus and unknowingly transmitted it to other people.

All in all, the second wave of the virus descended and it claimed lives with no discrimination of age, color, gender, religion, or affiliation.

It's worth emphasizing that the second wave was far more ferocious than the first. Furthermore, this iteration of the virus particularly targeted young adults, unlike the first wave. This incidence puzzled the doctors and other medical practitioners. Many diseases follow the "U-wave" while inflicting and killing people. That is, most diseases cause the deaths of many very young children and many very old people, but very few people who are in the prime of their lives. Yet, the second wave of the Spanish Flu caused the deaths of many such young people, astonishing everyone as it was well-established in 1918 that young people typically had the strongest immune systems. It was thought that these young people should have been fairly resistant to the flu.

Yet, what people did not know was the Spanish flu's second iteration attacked the body more brutally and strategically. The victims developed signs of mild flu just a few hours after contracting the virus. The symptoms would then escalate to full-blown misery, characterized by skin turning blue, difficulty breathing, and pneumonia-like symptoms. Upon performing post-mortems of the flu's victims, doctors observed that the victims' lungs were filled with fluid. This phenomenon meant that the patients had literally drowned in fluids produced by their own bodies. The lungs would also be stiff and displayed lesions.

The doctors tried to explain this strange phenomenon, claiming that these lesions were caused by the chemicals used during the war. Their explanation was easily accepted as the truth because the lesions were mainly observed in young people who were soldiers.

It was not until some decades later that this phenomenon was correctly understood as cytokine explosion. Cytokines are fluids released by the body's immune system to combat specific antigens in the body. The ability of the young adults' bodies to produce cytokines quickly and effectively should have worked to their advantage. During the first wave of the pandemic, the young adults' bodies had recognized and combatted the virus successfully, and after doing so, their immune systems retained a "memory" of the virus. This immune memory is specifically made from the recognition of the major components of the virus. Therefore, it is essential to understand that the virus that caused the second wave of the pandemic resulted from the mutation of the first virus.

So when the second iteration of the virus arrived, the immune system that had a memory of the first virus would therefore mistake the second virus for the first one. The immune system would then deploy "materials" for combatting the virus that caused the first wave, which were not effective in vanquishing the mutated virus. Unfortunately, it was these mechanisms that ended up destroying the body altogether. The cytokines that were so effective in fighting the virus of the first wave caused people to literally drown in their own lungs during the second wave.

17

In the end, the mutation caused the second wave of the Spanish flu to claim more lives than the first. In the US, 195,000 people perished in the month of October 1918 alone. In addition, some cities, such as Philadelphia, lost 748 people per 100,000 people during this second wave.

The second wave was so devastating, people thought the pandemic couldn't get any worse. However, the pandemic was far from over because the second wave was followed by a third wave. Though this wave was milder than the second, it carried on up to 1920. The third wave also exhibited a "U-wave" in terms of the victims it claimed, similar to the first wave. The third wave also hit Australia and Japan due to the soldiers who had returned from war. The wave then worked its way back to Europe, Africa, and the Americas.

Infecting 500 million people and claiming the lives of up to 100 million people, the Spanish flu is a pandemic that cannot be ignored. We have to seek to understand it as much as we can. Though we can never change the past, but there are always lessons we can learn from and apply to the present day, especially to our current experience with the coronavirus pandemic.

The Spanish Flu in Europe

Europe was among the first continents to be walloped by the 1918 pandemic. The disease may have been brought to Europe in two ways. In one theory, American soldiers who fought on the Allies' side during the first world war may have transmitted the virus to other soldiers and civilians. Another theory has been proposed by National Geographic that the Chinese laborers might have transmitted the disease to Europeans. They might have carried the disease from northern China to Canada and, eventually, to Europe. Since the media in Spain was neutral and not censored, Spanish media were the first party to report on the pandemic in detail. As a result, the flu was named the Spanish flu even though it did not originate from Spain.

In the United Kingdom, it was believed that soldiers returning from France were the carriers of the deadly virus. During the first wave of the pandemic, most of these soldiers suffered from mild flu symptoms. In fact, doctors called the disease the "three-day flu" or "three-day fever." These symptoms included fever, headache, sore throat, and loss of appetite. Altogether, the first wave was manageable for many soldiers, and even those who contracted it could easily undergo treatment using home remedies. Soldiers were believed to have contracted the disease due to unsanitary living conditions and from being in the trenches, which were no better than the camps.

At the end of the war, more soldiers returned to the United Kingdom by train.

They were oblivious of the fact that they were carriers of the virus that would comprise the second wave of the Spanish Flu pandemic. Consequently, the flu spread fast throughout the country like a wildfire. It spread from the railway stations to the city centers, to the suburbs, and eventually to rural areas.

The United Kingdom was not the only country that felt the venom of the pandemic. In Switzerland, people experienced their fair share of misery. It all started in early July 1918 when almost 70% of soldiers at the borders fell ill. The soldiers' commanders then decided to send the ill soldiers home, hoping they would recover and report back to work. Little did they know that this was the beginning of a raging disease that would eventually devastate the country.

When the soldiers went home, they were just mildly sick, so there was no cause for alarm. Even people who contracted the disease from them would be down for a few days, and then they would recover. This marked the first wave of the Spanish flu in Switzerland. But in September, people started falling ill again. This time, the flu was killing victims without delay. The victims would typically die just a few hours after contracting the disease. They would essentially suffocate to death, suffering from extreme pain. Their skin would turn blue due to lack of oxygen in their bodies, a condition known as cyanosis. The patients would also produce a blood-stained froth from their nose and mouth, obviously a distressing sight.

The most frightening fact was that there was no intervention that could save the victims' lives because the disease worked at lightning speed.

The Spanish flu claimed many lives in Switzerland. However, young men between 15-40 years old were the primary victims. This was partially due to their reluctance to follow physical distancing rules. For instance, they failed to adhere to the distancing rules that were established in military camps, brothels, and taverns when the pandemic became obvious. Therefore, these young men contracted the disease more often than women and the condition took a significant toll on them.

The disease caused the deaths of about 25,000 people in the country, while half the population was infected. The third wave occurred at the end of 1918 and it was milder than the second wave. The third wave prompted authorities in some cities such as Geneva to convene in order to find a solution for the pandemic.

In Geneva, all schools were closed and public gatherings were prohibited. To an extent, these closures helped curb the spread of the disease. Yet, the third wave of the pandemic continued wreaking havoc up to 1920. The Spanish flu has been considered the greatest pandemic in Switzerland in the country's modern history. The pandemic had a significant impact on the country's social, economic, and political lives, which can still be felt today.

Interestingly, Spain was perceived as the country that

suffered the most due to the Spanish flu.

Again, this was a mistaken assumption because the neutral Spanish media reported all the havoc caused by the pandemic. Ironically, many Spaniards believed that they got the disease from France and called it the "French Flu." There was heavy railroad traffic between France and Spain due to the droves of Spanish and Portuguese workers moving to or from France. Though Spain remained neutral throughout World War I, the country was going through a tremendous economic crisis due to the profound classism in the country. Spain was also experiencing the most significant inflation rates since the 1800s, with industrial strikes arising every now and again. In a nutshell, the Spanish economy was terrible and the country's atmosphere was tense.

In May 1918, Spain started experiencing the flu. The media reported on a strange flu-like malady that was afflicting many people in Madrid. The spread of the first wave of the contagion was greatly facilitated by the San Isidro festivals that were going on. The festivities brought together mass gatherings of people. Thereafter, people started falling ill with a mild disease, which mostly claimed the lives of small children, the elderly, and those with preexisting health conditions. But on May 28th, King Alfonso, the Spanish prime minister, and a number of cabinet members all fell ill. This spate of deaths showed people that the disease could infect and kill people of any social class, age, or gender.

In September 1918, another wave of the virus struck Spain. At first, the cases were isolated to certain regions. For instance, people would call it the Lorca Epidemic.

The Spaniards would even make fun of the disease, calling it El Mal de Moda (the disease of fashion) or the Naples Soldier. Little did they know that the disease would turn into a living nightmare in just a few weeks. During this second wave, as in so many other parts of the world, the young people in their prime were the most affected and they died in droves. When people would attend ceremonies, they would all fall ill and die overnight. Whole families would die at once, businesses collapsed, schools and universities shut down, and life as people knew it came to a standstill.

People in Spain frantically tried to seek solutions to cure this life-threatening malady. Doctors seemed to be utterly helpless in the face of this pandemic. Furthermore, most doctors, nurses, and other caretakers lost their lives while struggling to save those of the victims. Most people in the medical field were also greatly overworked due to the tremendous number of people stricken by the virus. Nothing seemed to deter the pandemic that appeared determined to kill all on its path.

As human efforts proved to be futile time and again, people turned to other sources for a solution. For instance, a bishop of the Catholic Church claimed that the pandemic was a punishment from God due to the sins committed by many. Clergy went so far as to recommend that people hold more church services for repentance and redemption.

During these services, people would gather, pray, and sing. As a part of their worship, they kissed the statues of some saints.

Despite their intentions, these gathering practices accelerated the spread of the disease, causing even more widespread suffering and death. In the town of Zamora, for example, mortality rates were among the highest in the whole of Spain. Zamora's people held several church services per day to repent for their "sins and lack of gratitude", which regrettably drew the pandemic to them like a moth to a flame.

The pandemic continued to inflict the Spaniards and affect their daily lives in immense ways. For instance, the delivery of goods by post was no longer possible due to the threat of contracting the disease from parcels. Schools were closed and some mass gatherings were prohibited. However, the churches remained open, and this ruling provided excellent conditions for the further propagation of the virus and obstructed the other efforts to curb the disease's spread. Civil authorities attempted to stop the church gatherings, but the bishop rebuked them for undue interruption of the church. Therefore, daily church services were held with an even larger multitude of people who were seeking solace from God during this time of sorrow. For its part, the Catholic Church preached that the pandemic was God's will and only God could deliver the people. In the church's view, the pandemic would come to an end not because of any human effort, but because of God's grace and mercy. At times, a common prayer called pro tempora pestilentia ("for the times of Pestilence") was offered. It highlighted the need for God to save people from the apparent plague and famine.

The third wave of the Spanish flu started in January 1919 and carried on to 1920. As previously mentioned, this wave was generally milder than the second wave. It mostly affected the geographical areas that were affected by the first wave and spared those areas that had been affected by the second wave.

The Spanish flu caused such a widespread demise of people that it caused a negative net population growth. In 1918, a total of 147,114 people died due to the disease. The contagion claimed 21,235 lives in 1919 and 17,285 in 1920. The second wave of the pandemic caused 75% of the deaths and was, definitively, the deadliest wave.

The disease spread to Portugal from Spain. The disease had devastating effects as with all the other regions it hit. However, one unique feature of the flu in Portugal was presence of the "safe villages." These villages were remote regions, mainly in the mountainous areas of Portugal, and they included some of the islands off the coast. These regions were independent long before the pandemic started. When the Spanish flu came into the picture, the villages isolated themselves and had few, if any, Spanish cases. As a result, even though many parts of Portugal were affected, as happened in so many other countries, its safe villages emerged from the flu somewhat better off than most other regions of the country. The majority of Portugal, however, suffered a great deal from the pandemic. In most cities, hundreds of people died.

In addition, the pandemic took aim at France. How the contagion got into France is disputed to this day.

It is thought that American soldiers who were carriers of the virus spread it to the French army and French civilians. Also, there were Indo-Chinese workers at French factories who could also have been carriers. But regardless of its provenance, the virus caused utter devastation in France.

The first cases in France were reported from the 3rd Army in Villers-Sur-Coudun and also in the training field at Fere-Briange between the dates of April 10th-20th, 1918. Another account attests that the virus broke out in an American camp based in the Bordeaux region of France. In its first wave, as in most other countries, the flu widely manifested itself as a mild and manageable disease. It was characterized by fever and other standard flu-like symptoms.

But after the Battle of the Somme, about 100 military men at the Etaples Military Camp fell ill. The Etaples Camp was a camp with some 100,000 troops who were either active or injured. However, the camp had only 24 sanatoriums. The doctors were quickly overwhelmed by the soldiers who fell prey to the contagion. During the second wave of the disease, the soldiers would contract the disease and die within hours. French people called the disease "la grippe" because the patients suffocated and died. The condition also had a visual sign: purple spots on the cheekbones. These spots were indicative that one had the disease and was most likely to die. For this reason, the French called the disease the Purple Death.

The disease caused utter despair mainly because it killed the young and healthy, leaving the French to have a shortage of healthy soldiers during the war. Likewise, people who worked in industries such as factories were also primarily young people at the prime of their lives. The scourge killed many of them, and for this reason, France's productivity was hampered, leading to a direct and detrimental impact on its economy.

Italy was also participating in World War I when the Spanish flu struck. Its people were severely impoverished, sick, and malnourished, and this contributed to the spread of the pandemic in the country. The Spanish flu first appeared in Italy in April 1918, and by 1920, it had claimed over 600,000 lives. During the second wave of the pandemic, about 100 people perished per day in Italy.

Throughout the European continent, the pandemic wreaked devastation on all people regardless of their social class, political affiliation, religion, or creed. People who were poor and lived in slums were significantly affected by the disease, but the virus did not spare prominent leaders of the time. King Alfonso of Spain died from the contagion, as did his prime minister and some cabinet members. The virus also afflicted the German Kaiser Wilhelm and claimed the lives of Austrian writers Egon Schiele and Gustav Klimt.

Guillaume Apollinaire, a French writer, and Hubert Parry, an English writer, also died of the scourge.

Europe was already in a crisis when the Spanish flu pandemic occurred. The continent was facing an enormous threat at that period—a global war. Its people had already experienced severe losses during World War I. In addition, medics were overwhelmed because, in addition to dealing with the pandemic victims, they were also treating injured soldiers. In short, the contagion was just another negative development. As bizarre as it may sound today, in Britain, people were asked to avoid speaking of the pandemic for as long as they could. The government wanted to avoid killing the "war morale." Thus, British people focused on the war because the outcome of the war would give them a new position on global politics and the economy.

In the meantime, doctors worked around the clock, trying to find a cure or vaccine for the pandemic. However, their efforts proved futile because they were mistakenly looking for a solution to Pfeiffer's bacillus instead of the influenza virus. However, not all their efforts were in vain because the field of medicine advanced in several ways. A step forward is always better than two steps backward, as the saying goes. Therefore as the forgotten pandemic comes back into the picture, there are ample lessons we can draw from it. Specifically, from the different responses of the various countries coping with it, we learn a great deal about preparedness and disaster management.

The Spanish Flu In America

Despite being called the Spanish flu, the 1918 pandemic could very well have originated in the US. The first recorded cases of the disease came from Camp Funston, a military base in Kansas. By now, we are already familiar with the story of how Mr. Gitchell, the camp cook, presented to the camp's clinic with a "bad flu" and how, by the evening, many more people at the camp presented with the same complaint. However, what we have not yet discussed is that since it was springtime at Camp Funston, there were about 17 species of birds that were migrating. The virus that caused the 1918 pandemic is thought to have originated from birds, then proceeded to infect pigs and hogs, and then finally spread to humans. While jumping from one species to the next, the virus mutated to become lethal and vicious. One characteristic trait of viruses is that they mutate, and while mutating, they develop new features that render the host's immune system unable to recognize them. In this manner, the mutated viruses enter the body and establish themselves without being detected by the immune system. Furthermore, even when they are detected, the immune system may mistake the viruses for other pathogens, thereby making the immune system's elimination efforts self-destructive to the body as a whole rather than protective.

When the disease was first reported in January 1918, it was described as a mild disease that was fairly insignificant because, despite infecting many people, the mortality rate was initially very low.

In Britain at that time, for instance, 10,318 soldiers were

admitted to the sickbay, but only four of them died. This circumstance prompted people to conclude that the sickness was too mild to be considered as influenza. However, it spread from Camp Funston to almost 30 other military camps throughout the US as well as to the civilian population. As the "doughboys" were sent to Europe to fight during the First World War, they carried the disease with them. Before even reaching Europe, some men had already perished due to the disease. Though the disease had previously been considered mild, a local physician named Miner Loring blew the whistle that there was unusual "influenza" activity that year. Loring's announcement was considered the first alarm of the 1918 pandemic in the US. The first wave did not cause widespread death of many people, due to the mildness of the symptoms, and many patients were misdiagnosed as having meningitis.

As the days went by, the disease became normalized. It was called the "three-day fever" and a couple of other names that depicted it as a weak disease. In fact, by July 1918, some media houses reported that the epidemic was almost coming to an end. Moreover, in Britain, some journalists plainly stated that the pandemic was over. These statements evoke the image of a tsunami first sucking water from the shore, leaving it clear and calm, before forcing out a destructive tower of water that no one can survive. This image was precisely the case with the pandemic.

The first sign of the resurgence of the Spanish flu was in Switzerland, and it arrived in a particularly vicious form. In August 1918, an American navy intelligence officer based in

Switzerland wrote a report that stated he was witnessing a disease that was savaging the Swiss population. He described it as the Black Plague or the Spanish Gripe. The report was addressed to the US government as secret and confidential. In just a matter of days, the second wave started ravaging the US, commencing in a military base known as Camp Devens, located near Boston. This camp had 45,000 soldiers and its hospital facility could accommodate up to 1,200 patients, a good facility by the standards of that time.

September 7th, 1918 began like a typical day to most soldiers at Camp Devens. An excellent day to recruit, train, and maybe send more doughboys to Europe in the ongoing World War. However, a soldier was admitted at the hospital, and he was restless, delirious, and screaming in pain.

To the hospital staff, the only infection that could possibly manifest as his symptoms was meningitis. Meningitis causes inflammation of the meninges of the brain and this may result in brain damage, which eventually may lead to loss of brain function. The next day, a dozen more men were admitted with the same alarming symptoms—hysterical, screaming, and kicking—and this further raised the doctors' eyebrows. But this was just the beginning, as the following day, even more men were admitted in the same condition. Only then did the doctors change the diagnosis from meningitis to influenza.

You may be wondering how the physicians could change their minds at the snap of a finger. We need to understand

31

that viruses, bacteria, or fungi can cause meningitis. Whatever the causative agent, the disease is mild to moderately communicable. Therefore, the rate at which the disease was spreading ruled out the possibility of its being meningitis. Panic rose in the camp. An army report was released and it reported that influenza was exploding throughout the camp. More soldiers fell ill with each passing day. At the height of the pandemic, 1,537 soldiers reported ill and were admitted to the camp's hospital.

Needless to say, the hospital at Camp Devens was overwhelmed. The facility was already experiencing a shortage of medical practitioners. More than half of the US's doctors and nurses had been shipped off to Europe to care for the injured during the war. The virulence of the disease was so high that it caused the demise of the patient long before the physicians' intervention could work. The rate at which the disease spread was also mind-blowing. Therefore, the doctors and nurses were overworked, overwhelmed, and clearly at a loss on what to do. We should not forget that they, too, were not immune to the disease and a good number of them died at the line of duty, trying desperately to save the lives of people from the ravages of the Spanish flu.

In the US, patients presented with flu-like symptoms that would escalate to shortness of breath, which would lead to the complete inability to breathe.

Patients would then develop strange mahogany spots over the cheekbones. These spots became the most dangerous sign because from that point, patients would turn blue (cyanosis). Cyanosis would begin from the tips of the ears to the whole face. The patients would then produce the alarming bloodstained froth from their mouth and nose.

In some cases, blood would ooze out of patients' ears and noses. This development deeply puzzled the physicians and a physician in Chicago began to suggest that the disease was new. Upon doing autopsies, the doctors were surprised to find that the lungs of the patients were filled with fluid and were as hard as stone. They were alarmed to see that patients literally suffocated in their own lungs.

The contagion, as in many parts of the world, claimed the lives of young Americans in the prime of their lives. A cloud of despondency hung over the hospital at Camp Devens. At some point, the camp's hospital refused to take in more patients because there was no longer room for them, much less medical staff to service the new patients. Devastation hung in the air, with the hospital reporting about 100 deaths per day. The saddest and most frightening aspect was that the patients would come in with mild flu symptoms only for the symptoms to rapidly escalate, and, within the next few hours, they would be pronounced dead.

Hospital management was also struggling with the disposal of the mounting number of dead bodies.

So many people perished that the hospital had to arrange for mass burial. They made these arrangements as hastily as possible to reduce the risk of people contracting the illness from the corpses.

The disease did not stop at Camp Devens and in just a matter of weeks, almost the whole of the US was experiencing the wrath of the scourge. The young, the old, the poor the rich, the powerful, and the helpless alike fell prey to it. From Boston, the disease spread to Philadelphia. In early September, a ship from Boston docked in Philadelphia, and as soon as the ship docked, two sailors died of a flu-like illness. By this time, people in Philadelphia had gotten wind of the occurrences in Boston. In no time, inhabitants had already heard about the two dead sailors and were afraid that the contagion had set foot in the city. To calm citizens, city authorities claimed that the sailors died from the old-fashioned "grip" and not the already infamous Spanish flu. But the following day, fourteen sailors died from the same disease. Still, Philadelphia authorities once again reassured people that the Spanish flu did not cause the situation and that they would nip the disease in the bud. At this point in history, the US was already facing a major crisis that was the ongoing World War. Therefore, just as in Britain, Americans were prohibited from spreading messages that would bring down war morale.

This attitude became even more lethal than the contagion when the US entered the war. The president demanded that the spirit of ruthless brutality be part of the nation's every fiber.

A law was even passed prohibiting people from uttering, printing, writing, or publishing profanities along with disloyal and treacherous statements about the US government. This law also forbid any activities that involved urging, advocating, or inciting the curtailing of anything that helped in the prosecution of the war. This law was known as the Sedition Act.

Failure to adhere to Sedition Act would lead to serving a jail term of 20 years. Fear is said to be one of the most effective ways to control a population, and the Sedition Act instilled fear in everyone. Therefore, people stopped talking about the lethal pandemic despite that its brutality was right in front of them. Some people, especially sycophants, would even go to the extent of reporting those who attempted to talk about the flu and its effects. Such people were said to be spreading pessimistic lies. Despite that the pandemic was continuing to show its grim face to the public, public health officers continued to lie in order to maintain the spirit of war. What other choice did they have in a country that convicted those that spread "pessimistic lies, cries for peace, or anyone belittling the country's effort to win the war"?

By September 26th 1918, many military camps across the country were struggling to deal with an increasing number of infected soldiers on top of the soldiers who were already dead. For this reason, all the camps halted their drafting process despite the need for soldiers in the battlefield. The majority of the states also canceled their mass celebrations.

However, the city of Philadelphia was reluctant to do cancel celebrations and mass gatherings, and on September 28th, they held the largest Liberty Loan Parade ever held in the country.

The purpose of this parade was to demand funds for the war. The parade was held despite the protests against it from doctors and medical practitioners. Doctors had written to media houses, urging them to speak out about the dangers of convening amidst a pandemic. Yet, none of the newspapers wrote about it, probably due to fear of suffering the consequences of the Sedition Act. Some doctors tried to write letters to the public via the newspapers, but none of them would be published. As for civilians, most of them attended the Liberty Loan Parade despite witnessing the disease laying waste to their fellow citizens. This event surely evokes the saying that common sense is not common to all.

So the Liberty Loan Parade was held with people out and about chanting slogans and seemingly feeling invincible. The incubation period for influenza virus is 2-3 days, and true to that timeline, people started falling ill two days after the parade. At last, the city's mayor conceded that the disease that was said to be present only in military camps had now spread to the civilian population, but lies were still in place. The mayor urged the citizens not to panic over exaggerated reports, but the fact was that the Sedition Act would prevent anyone from exaggerating.

Being in power meant that the media was on the mayor's side. The newspaper *The Inquirer* had a headline that read "Scientific Nursing Halting Epidemic." This headline was a blatant lie because there were few nurses in the country at that time, with many of the country's medical practitioners having been conscripted to help during the war. The few nurses who were available were either sick or overworked, and unfortunately, much of the country did not approve of the African-American nurses who were available to work in the hospitals. But as more people fell ill and perished, the mayor gave in. He gave orders to close all schools and banned all public gatherings. However, it was too little too late, as the contagion had infected all of Philadelphia, making Philadelphia one of the most affected US cities of the pandemic.

At the peak of the pandemic's destruction, Philadelphia lost 793 people in one day. Managing the dead became too difficult because so many people were dying within a very short duration. The city morgue was designed to harbor only 50 people at a time, and now people were dying over ten times that capacity each day. On one particular day, the city's priests went down the empty streets, calling on people to bring out their dead loved ones. The priests would later dig mass graves and bury the corpses. Of all the people who died during this second wave of the Spanish flu, the most affected were the young people who died excruciating and terrifying deaths.

The pandemic was not only wreaking havoc in Philadelphia. In Arkansas, it leveled the people. In the hospital at Camp Pike, the pneumonia unit was completely overwhelmed. There were rows and rows of cots with patients who seemed to get worse with each passing minute. The doctors were at a loss. Never had they witnessed so much death at the camp. As if oblivious to the situation, a newspaper named *The Gazette* published that the pandemic was the "same old Spanish grip with the same old chills and fever." The more people who hungered for truth, the deeper the US government continued to bury it. But people were edging closer and closer to their breaking point.

The Spanish flu was cunning in many ways, but the most astonishing thing about it is that it found a way to reach certain Alaskan communities. Though the pandemic had touched nearly the entire world, the state of Alaska was among the most unlikely to be affected by the pandemic because many Alaskan communities were aloof to any form of interaction with the outside world. The people in these communities had not heard about the contagion that was ravaging the world.

But on July 4th, 1918, a ship arrived at Bristol Bay in Alaska. Three children with weak, feverish bodies landed on the beach. Aboard the same ship were the bodies of two dead men. The residents of Bristol Bay were astonished, having been completely unaware of the destruction that was happening in other villages. The children were taken to a hospital run by a salmon company.

After they got well, a search team was directed to a village further upstream.

The search team could not believe what they saw in the village. Devastation was a mere understatement of the situation. Dead bodies were lying everywhere. In some places, they would find stray dogs scavenging on the dead bodies. Death had reigned terror on the villages and what was left of the villagers was just a faint shadow of their former selves. There was no activity whatsoever; no hunting, no fishing, no gathering, and absolutely no children playing around, filling the air with their sweet melodies.

Yet in that particular village, the search team encountered a group of people who were alive. They were feeble and sickly. They told the search team of how they had witnessed the other villagers seemingly drop dead while walking around. They recounted how the disease had wiped off the village's population at breakneck speed. If the search team thought they had seen it all, this was just the beginning, as numerous other villages in Alaska experienced the very same catastrophe. Most villages were entirely wiped out.

The search team had to dig mass graves in most of the villages in order to properly dispose of the bodies. The Alaskan population had the highest mortality rate per capita. This means that though the Alaskan population was sparse, 90% of its people were infected by the disease.

Speculation has been made to determine why the pandemic hit Alaska particularly hard, especially in certain remote villages. These villages were miles and miles away from any other village. Therefore, the village inhabitants did not encounter many disease-causing microorganisms, so their immunity was low. Their lack of immunity and exposure to disease were likely the reasons why the Spanish flu took an incredibly heavy toll on the people.

The affliction of the Spanish Flu on the Alaskan community could be considered a blessing in disguise, as bizarre as it may sound. The extremely cold conditions of this region preserved the bodies of the victims. As a result, in 1972, a medical student named John Hultin went to an Inuit community, where he asked for permission to unearth and examine the frozen bodies of several Spanish flu victims. Later, in the 1990s, this research led to the determination of the causative agent of the deadliest pandemic in modern history. The Spanish flu pandemic also opened up the remote Alaskan communities to the outside world, bringing about new developments in its society.

Overall, the Spanish flu pandemic affected the whole of the US and it had a resounding effect on almost every inch of the country. However, there is still an Alaskan community that puzzles scientists to date: the Egegak Community. The scourge did not afflict this community at all. Among the places that were untouched by this pandemic were walled schools and asylums, along with remote villages and islands. These areas were called the "escape communities."

The reason why these communities were spared from the scourge was because they had no contact whatsoever with the outside world.

The Spanish flu in the US highlights so many lessons for us to learn, the most important of which is the need to be truthful at all times. It is better to face any circumstance fully aware of it, however horrific it may be, rather than trying to move forward oblivious of the lies holding us back.

The Spanish Flu in Africa

The global outbreak of the 2020 coronavirus pandemic has now made the term "pandemic" a common word in our daily lives. Among the old and young, rural and urban, civilized and uncivilized, developed and developing countries, we have all felt major distress caused by the coronavirus pandemic.

This outbreak inspires us to look at similar experiences in the past. Within the recent 20th century, a similar pandemic, if not an even more disastrous one, brought the world to a standstill. Characterized by rapid spread and progression of the disease, the outbreak of the Spanish flu led to the deaths of many individuals in almost all corners of the globe.

In this section, I will delve into the pandemic as it hit the African continent. Much of the recorded and available information covers the impact the pandemic had on Europe and the Americas. The sparse information available on the pandemic's impact on Africa will be used to provide details. But first, a brief history and pathogenesis of the Spanish flu is crucial.

The Spanish flu outbreak of 1918-1920 hit its likely peak of the epidemic in Etaples, a military camp in northern France. It was not Spain, as was widely publicized.

The first victims of the disease were US soldiers in March 1918 at a military base in Kansas. Within the first three months of the outbreak, the flu had widely spread among the European countries as the soldiers moved around during the First World War. The causative agent is the virus H1N1, which is of avian origin. The disease majorly attacked the respiratory system. Some of the clinical presentations were acute cyanosis, blood in vomit, and a hacking cough.

Most of the infected individuals died of acute respiratory distress syndrome (ARDS) following infection. Being an airborne disease, the flu's spread was so rapid that within the period of 1918-1919, an estimated third of the world's population had been infected, with close to 50 million deaths. The disease was especially brutal as it took special aim at those at the prime ages of their lives, with most deaths occurring among those in the age bracket of 24-34 years. These deaths were in stark contrast to the 2020 coronavirus pandemic that has seen most deaths among the elderly and infants. Therefore, the impact of the Spanish flu pandemic was truly terrifying.

The pathogenicity of the Spanish flu virus remained unclear until the late 1990s when advancements had been made in technological and medical fields. At the time when the flu broke out, most of the information on the causative agent and the virulence of the virus remained unknown for a long period. These delays in learning could be blamed on both poor technology and lack of sufficient knowledge in the medical field as compared to today. In later years, the

Spanish flu was found to be an RNA influenza virus.

As the disease broke out, most of the deaths that occurred were due to pneumonia. Secondary bacterial pneumonia led to the loss of lives of most individuals. This was largely due to lack of antibiotics to counter the bacterial agents and partly due to poor health-service provisions. Viral pneumonia was also implicated in the manifestations of the patients who presented with the disease. The course of infection lasted for five days or less. Extensive destruction of the lungs was typically observed with a characteristic hemorrhagic exudate in them. Extensive edema ensued following the collapse of the lungs.

On matters regarding the virulence of the 1918 virus, it is considered worse than the 21st-century novel swine-origin H1N1 influenza virus that broke out in 2009. Surprisingly, most of the people survived the swine-flu pandemic despite that it was H1N1. This is due to the innate and adaptive immune factors in our bodies. However, the millions of deaths seen during the Spanish flu crisis can be attributed to its widespread infections around the world. The entire globe was affected by it.

In the African continent, communities were initially hardly hit by the pandemic. Within the first six months of the surge of the pandemic in 1918, 2% of Africa's population had succumbed to death from the disease. The mortality rate is estimated to have been close to 15% during the pandemic.

Among the countries that were hardest hit were South Africa, Nigeria, and Sierra Leone. South Africa was the worst hit nation in the entire continent, with close to 5% of South Africa's population succumbing to death. In western Africa, the route of entry of the disease was Freetown. Therefore, it is not surprising that it was the hardest hit spot in the region, with 4% of its population dying of the pandemic. It is also important to note that Freetown had been a center for freed slaves in Africa.

The Spanish flu was characterized by a short incubation period of 1-2 days. Medical facilities during the time of the outbreak were overwhelmed. The spread of this pandemic was seen in three waves, as seen elsewhere in the world. The first wave hit the northern parts of Africa in the earlier months of 1918. The second wave hit sub-Saharan Africa, which had been largely spared during the first wave. The entry of the infections during this wave was through the seaports of western Africa. Countries hit during this time included Ghana, Nigeria, and Sierra Leone. Later, the calamity spread to the southern parts of Africa. The third wave hit during the month of December 1918.

Several factors contributed to the spread of the pandemic in Africa. One major factor was World War I, which was occurring at the time of the calamity. Troops and laborers were often being transported from battlefields, and to and from the military camps. This movement promoted the spread of the virus. Warships that docked in coastal cities such as Cape Town, Mombasa, and Freetown acted as key entry routes of the Spanish flu into the African continent.

Urban centers along the coastline often served as trade and transport centers. Railway lines and water transport via major rivers connected these urban towns with the interior communities. Mining activities were taking place in the rural areas that required ferrying of the mined products to the seaports. As such, it was through movement to and from the coastal towns into the urban areas that facilitated the economic activities, which in turn enabled the spread of the disease to rural areas.

Another factor that promoted the spread of the pandemic was tension and fear among individuals. As the virus hit coastal towns, the inhabitants were gripped with fear of losing their lives. This resulted in widespread migration from the coastal urban centers into the villages. This mass movement of people caused widespread infection across the continent. In Ethiopia, for example, the pandemic took out the lives of the few medical personnel that could help fight the disease. This loss of life resulted in increased spread and deaths across the nation.

The impact the global pandemic had on Africa cannot be underestimated. Though all the continents were affected, Africa, the cradle of humankind, was not left unscathed. The disease hit the region when most of its nations and kingdoms were under colonial rule. At the same time, there was World War I. It is worth noting that in that period, the African continent was backward in terms of infrastructure and development. Also, under the colonial powers, the natives were deprived of freedom.

Even though there is insufficient historical data on the impact of the Spanish flu on African nations, some information can be obtained from colonial records and other records passed down through informal reports or stories. In Kenya, for example, the disease is thought to have hit the nation around September 1918 when a ship from India docked at the Kenyan coast. Moreover, the spread into African rural areas was heightened by the return of frontline African soldiers who had been conscripted to fight in World War I as the common-service unit then known as the "carrier corps." A military organization that had acquired African natives for the war resettled the soldiers into their various native lands, thereby hastening the spread of the virus. Deaths were seen among people of both Black and white race. The infection spared none. Inadequate access to better healthcare increased the mortality rate, especially among the natives in comparison with the privileged white settlers.

In Kenya, information regarding the disease was reported mainly through the provincial administration to the British colonial authorities. Village elders often conducted meetings popularly known as "barazas" to brief the community on the disease and gather any vital information on deaths. This sparse data can be retrieved from these colonial records. As stated earlier, the flu spared none. It hit both whites and African Black natives alike.

Colonial authorities stipulated certain health interventions to help curb community spread. Personal hygiene, social distancing, and medical treatment were the major interventions. Healthy individuals were to distance themselves from infected individuals. Prophylactic measures, such as gargling with potassium permanganate and oral quinine, were provided to those that could access hospital care. Unfortunately, most of the native Africans could not cope with the provided regulations or, rather, the information never reached them. Thus, the spread was not curbed as much as expected. At the same time, as people moved to escape from infected people, they further spread the disease across the country. Records of deaths from the period are not clear on how many deaths were from the Spanish flu, as most of the data on the pandemic was acquired through informal means.

The Spanish flu pandemic had certain social impacts on society. For instance, South Africa had both white occupants and Black occupants of native African origin. The outbreak in that country led to the segregation of the Blacks by the privileged whites. Thus arose "Sanitation Syndrome." The white community started fearing that Blacks were spreading the infection—consequently, the then government, which was dominated by white colonialists legally enforced racial segregation. The enforcement of racial segregation was characterized by brutality toward the natives, creating animosity between the groups, with Blacks being denigrated.

A notable impact was the loss of many lives. As a result of the death toll, many children were left orphans. Individuals who died in their prime left their children without someone to take care of them. This increased suffering among the African people. John Spears, in his writings about "Bechuanaland", elaborates on the suffering that these orphans had to go through to meet their daily basic needs. Most of the communities came to understand the flu as an airborne disease that spread through the breath. There was then the coining of the term "fierce breath." Segregation of infected family members became the only option. People had to flee the fierce breath of loved ones in order to protect themselves. Such actions impaired the social well-being of the community.

Throughout the African continent, the pandemic resulted in lifestyle changes. Customs and practices that were previously considered immutable abruptly changed. In Ghana, for example, there was a switching of gender roles. In Ghana, the infection had largely affected pregnant women and mothers. These deaths left motherless children with their fathers, forcing the fathers to take on roles previously assigned to women in the prevailing culture. These roles included fetching firewood, cooking, and feeding the children. The death of pregnant women also resulted in the demise of the fetuses.

Likewise, in Nigeria, a country with people who had once dismissed the plant cassava as part of their diet, adopted the plant as one of its staple foods.

One reason for this about-face was that cultivation of cassavas did not require too much agricultural labor, as it could be cultivated just once. Moreover, it took several periods for the plants to grow. In times of crisis, the cassava plant became the savior to many from hunger. In addition, during the pandemic, the deaths of the young and those in their prime resulted in the loss of human labor to carry out much of the farming.

The African economic sector was also not spared in the pandemic's turmoil. Gloom covered the land, not just from the loss of loved ones, but also due to the loss of many communities' source of livelihood. In Zimbabwe (then called Southern Rhodesia), a British colony in the southern part of Africa, there was a closure of gold mines. The Globe and Phoenix Gold Mine in Umvuma closed down due to loss of human labor to run the mining activities. The company failed to pick up again even by the pandemic's end, which brought Zimbabwe's economic life to a standstill.

Also, the return of soldiers who had gone to fight in World War I heralded the spread of the infection in more rural areas. However, most of the individuals who died at the start of the virus's spread in the African continent were soldiers. In Zambia, for instance, the flu largely took the lives of soldiers. The people, therefore, regarded the disease as a "war air." Later, with the spread from military camps, people scattered in the country were seeking isolation from the infected patients. This mass movement hastened the spread across the nation.

Many names were therefore coined to name the disease based on its fast spread. Stories were narrated to pass onto future generations regarding this great calamity. These stories passed down to younger generations are one of the major sources of information regarding the spread of the pandemic in Africa.

Notably, most of the Black African natives had previously regarded their European masters as superior. They had for a long period cherished their skin color and saw them as unique for that reason. Unlike them, the whites were close to gods. However, that narrative changed with the surge of the pandemic, when the natives saw their masters also being infected by the disease, falling sick, and even dying of the infection. The Africans who had been taken to fight in the war and survived the pandemic realized that Europeans were not gods, but just like them.

In the African colonial states, such as Namibia, the whites were not spared by the disease despite having access to better healthcare than the native Africans. In Sierra Leone, a British colony, the colonial records give information on the depths of the disaster in the land. The disease is believed to have been entered the country by a warship in Freetown. Much of the impact of the pandemic was experienced among the armed forces, prisons, and soldiers. This impact was due to the interaction between the soldiers and the inmates. In the rural areas of Sierra Leone, there was severe stigmatization of the infected persons. Some individuals were even chased out of their homes and left to die homeless.

Provision of good healthcare was unheard of in the country. Most of the native African patients died due to lack of healthcare access.

The colonial African governments adopted several measures to mitigate the impact and effect of the pandemic across the continent. Since the infection was airborne, large gatherings were banned throughout most of the countries. Social distancing became a normal routine amidst the pandemic. Groups in churches, schools, bars, and markets were abolished. Quarantine measures were imposed on the infected individuals and people entering the continent through seaports into the various countries. These measures would limit their contact with the healthy population.

The government campaigned for early communication by establishing lines of administration and communication. The village elders and community leaders were to act as a connection between medical authorities and the people on the ground level. This line of communication would facilitate what is known today as the "contact tracing" of infection by tracking infected individuals and their contacts. Another beneficial intervention was the setting up of temporary health facilities by volunteer groups within African nations, including South Africa and Nigeria. In Nigeria, there was also the adoption of house-to-house searches. Yet, this particular intervention proved to be unfruitful. In the city of Lagos, the Health Ordinance Mandate of 1917 gave medical authorities, who were largely comprised of white people, the power to access people's homes.

This became an intrusion into a community's space, and the intervention engendered fear, causing people to flee their homes into other areas. Consequently, the disease spread further. Lack of trust and communication between medical authorities and locals stalled the interventions. Most of the natives feared medicine as they saw it as a white man's poison.

In conclusion, the 20th century was characterized by many unfortunate events. First, there was World War I that created a hub for the rapid spread of the deadly disease popularly coined the Spanish flu. This virus with its high infection rate was able to sweep through the entire globe within three years. With its high mortality rate, an estimated 20-50 million people succumbed to death from the virus. The pandemic remains tainted in the minds of many people and historians. It brings to mind a world of the oneness that we ought to have as human beings in such situations. Some of the effects that the catastrophe wrought on the world included a sharp drop in food production, shortages of labor, and impoverishment of the social livelihood of human beings. Many children were orphaned, leading to their suffering and poverty.

As the world battles the 2020 pandemic of coronavirus, we can absorb a few lessons from these past disasters. From the Spanish flu outbreak, we have learned that all countries, despite their few minor differences, belong to one global community. In a bid to handle any catastrophe, the outbreak brought to our attention the importance of communication, which is one of the pillars of building trust and integrity.

As the people of one big global village, we had ought to

communicate on matters affecting us all and collectively share the burden. For example, actions should be made to tackle food security in case of any other future outbreaks.

Finally, we have learned that in handling a calamity, we ought to provide long-term measures to be sustained for a relatively long period that, for the Spanish Flu, could have prevented the second and even third waves of the outbreak.

The Spanish Flu in Asia

As the 1918 pandemic roamed throughout the world, it did not spare Asia. However, before we delve into how the Spanish flu affected Asia and its people, let us first learn about the types of influenza.

There are four types of the influenza virus that affect human beings: types A, B, C, and D. Only type A influenza has caused pandemics in history. The Spanish flu was caused by influenza of type A, the subtype H1N1, whereas the Avian Flu pandemic was caused by another type A influenza, the subtype H2N2. The Spanish flu was thought to have originated from Asia, particularly China. This origin theory derives from how in November 1917, in northern China, a flu-like illness afflicted numerous people. This illness caused death within a few hours after onset. Patients would suffer from cyanosis and produce a bloody froth from their mouths and noses. Does this sound familiar? These are the very same symptoms that victims of the Spanish flu had to endure, particularly in the second wave.

However, Chinese medical officials labeled the disease "winter sickness." Consequently, no quarantine measures were enforced and no travel restrictions were enabled, setting the stage for the propagation of the Spanish flu.

From northern China to other parts of the world, the Spanish flu wreaked unfathomable disaster, infecting almost half the world's population and claiming up to 100 million lives. In Asia, India is the country that was arguably the most affected by this contagion. The disease set foot in the country when a group of British soldiers docked in the city of Bombay.

Bombay was an overcrowded city, which provided the perfect conditions for the rapid spread of the disease. Like a bushfire, the disease spread far and wide to the Himalayas mountain ranges, along the Ganges River, and essentially to every part of the country.

India's people were totally unprepared for such a pandemic. India's healthcare system had been neglected by the British colonizers. As the majority of the country's native citizens were living in abject poverty, they were malnourished and this increased their susceptibility to the illness.

When the disease first struck Bombay, the natives were convinced that it was the British soldiers who brought this pestilence upon them. However, when the colonial government perceived that they could not control the disease, they blamed it on the natives. The British said that the pestilence was occurring due to the natives' unsanitary conditions, which provoked anger among the Indian natives.

The disease caused universal turmoil in India. Many people were afflicted by the disease and the few available hospitals were filled to the brim. This situation caused the Indian leaders to urge the people to try practicing home-care remedies. As if to add salt to the wound, a famine struck India during this time. Malnourished and poverty-stricken, the majority of India's population fell prey to the unforgiving pandemic, and most of the victims perished.

Leaders and civilians alike were affected by the disease. The legendary Mahatma Gandhi contracted the disease. It caused him such excruciating torture that he had to consume a liquid diet. One newspaper in India wrote, "Gandhi's life is not his anymore; it is in the hands of India." The Spanish flu clearly showed that the British government had neglected the lives of native Indians and were solely in India to benefit their own country. This conflict of interest caused so much fury among the Indians that it augmented their thirst for independence. The pandemic was a wake-up call for the Indian people to take charge of their resources.

Victims of the flu in India would suffer the typical host of symptoms: lack of oxygen, excruciating pain throughout the body, and would ooze bloodstained froth from their mouths and ears. Many people were infected just a few days after the Spanish flu arrived in India. No remedies seemed to work quickly enough to curb the disease and its spread. Also, at that time, most of India's population was not accustomed to Western medicine. Moreover, Western medicine didn't work on those who were using it. Death and destruction were everywhere. With the colonial government maintaining a hands-off policy, the Indian government took up the role of cautioning the people, informing them, and consoling them. This was one of the government's most significant steps in dispelling desolation from the hearts of the Indians. The country's newspapers urged the people to maintain proper sanitation, remain at home, and most importantly, not to worry too much about the pandemic.

For instance, the newspaper *The Times of India* wrote that people should stay indoors to avoid human contact. The newspaper also informed people that the disease was spread by secretions of the nose and mouth. With this information, people could at least try to avoid contracting this malady. Yet, the invisible grim reaper did not stop laying waste to the lives of the Indian population. The virus claimed up to 18 million lives. The prominent Indian poet Nerada lost his whole family.

Death was so widespread in India that there was not enough firewood to cremate the bodies of the deceased. Nerada wrote that people died within the blink of an eye and that the Ganges River was swollen with Indian bodies. The pandemic left India in a desolate state and the colonial government did not help the people in any way. The situation was dire until non-governmental organizations (NGOs) came to the people's aid. They helped treat the sick as well as cremate the bodies of those who were already dead. These NGOs also helped restore the working state of hospitals, which had been overwhelmed by the vast number of ill patients and many corpses. While the disease devastated India, the silver lining to all this destruction is that the Spanish flu gave the Indians a solid reason to fight for their independence. It was a wake-up call that only they, as the native Indian population, would genuinely care for their needs. They realized that the colonials were there to solely benefit themselves.

From India, we will move on to its neighbor, China. It has been previously stated that China could have been the origin of the scourge that became the Spanish flu. However, the effect of the disease on the Chinese people was somewhat milder than on the majority of the other parts of the world. This outcome seems to contrast with our expectations because, at the time, China was just a shadow of its current state as a global superpower. Back then, it was a country with middling economy and a feeble medical system by modern standards. Nonetheless, China managed to effectively and fairly efficiently control the pandemic. Another astonishing aspect about the pandemic in China is that while in other parts of the world, the pandemic claimed mainly the lives of adults between 15-40 years old, in China it mainly claimed the lives of those between 11-15 years old. Furthermore, the mortality rate was meager compared to the mortality rate in the Western world.

The first phase of the Spanish flu pandemic in China was well-observed by Dr. A Stanley, who was working in Shanghai. He described that the influenza first appeared at the end of May and lasted until June. In this phase, the flu caused mild symptoms such as headache, fever, muscle aches, and sore throat, all akin to a common cold. These patients also presented with erythema, leading some to confuse the flu with scarlet fever. However, between October and November, the flu had more severe symptoms and a higher number of casualties. These symptoms included bronchitis and pneumonia, which eventually led to the demise of a number of patients.

The number of patients also increased sharply during this phase. But against all odds, the death toll remained incredibly low.

However, in some villages, there was a relatively higher death toll, probably because of the lack of the village inhabitants' previous exposure to influenza. In these villages, there would be burials every day. Out of 200 inhabitants, about 40 of them would perish. The disease dealt a hard blow to these communities due to their lack of previous exposure to the disease.

Interestingly, traditional Chinese Medicine played a significant role in the management of the pandemic. In a world where Western medicine was still in its infancy, the Chinese were more comfortable practicing what they had known and perfected since time immemorial. Chinese medical practice had particularly emphasized how to deal with epidemics. In Chinese medicine, there were over 120 texts filled with details on handling outbreaks. According to these texts, the two main characteristics of outbreaks were that they occurred in many people (high infectiousness) regardless of age and that they manifested the same signs and symptoms (uniformity in the manifestation of symptoms). When it was obvious that the Spanish flu embodied these two characteristics, Chinese healthcare providers followed the age-old instructions on quarantine, social distancing, and practices of good hygiene. In addition, those who were infected were offered herbal remedies, and, against all odds, these remedies worked.

These herbal remedies included the very effective Mahuang Xingren Shingao, a concoction made by several renowned practitioners of traditional Chinese medicine.

In the end, China was the country with the highest recovery rate in the world, with a rate of 97% among men and 96% among women. The rate was higher in women probably because they were the primary caretakers of the ill, and this left most of them exposed to the disease.

Chinese anti-epidemic therapy has stood the test of time. It has given the Chinese an upper hand in managing epidemics and pandemics. As for their traditional remedies, they have proven to be effective against the disease in question. What is yet to be explained is whether these remedies are antiviral, if they boost immunity, or if they accomplish both—all in all, better half a loaf than no bread, as the saying goes. In other words, sometimes we don't need any savior—we are our own savior. For their part, the Chinese did not need external intervention to deal with the life-threatening disease.

In the ongoing coronavirus pandemic, individuals and countries are urged to look within to try to find a long-lasting solution. Sometimes nature reminds us that we are small systems that contribute to one colossal structure: the universe. Our contribution, no matter how little, may bring a tremendous change. China's example also reminds us not to lose our heritage while in pursuit of the modern.

Japan has suffered several pandemics in the past: the Asian flu, the Hong Kong flu, the Russian flu, among others. However, none of the plagues took a more significant toll on the country than Spanish flu. The first wave of the disease hit the country relatively late. This delay may be due to Japan's distance from Europe, where the disease struck first, or the geographical difficulty of accessing the island republic. According to medical records from several hospitals in Japan the first wave of the pandemic was relatively mild, presenting with signs of the typical flu. The Japanese referred to it as "Knabo Fever." Little did the people know that this seemingly benign disease would cause destruction that they had not witnessed in a long time.

Most of the information on the Spanish flu in Japan is based on data from hospitals. Most of the patients were members of the army—robust young men. The Tokyo First Army Hospital, which admitted mainly army members, provides medical records that document the pandemic. From January 1918 to September 1918, the hospital admitted several respiratory illness cases, including acute bronchitis, pneumonia, and influenza. According to its records, the mortality rates due to acute bronchitis and pneumonia were incredibly low, and for influenza, the rate was at 0%. People were oblivious that they were experiencing the first wave of the pandemic.

In November 1918, the number of influenza patients

shot to 109, and 8% of them would die. This marked the beginning of widespread destruction caused by the Spanish flu pandemic.

Patients who were admitted in November 1918 were violently ill. Most of them reported to the clinic with fever, chills, headaches, coughing, and muscle aches. In time, they would develop more severe symptoms and bacterial pneumonia, which eventually led to their demise. Doctors described their patients as having facial expressions that conveyed utter agony and misery. The patients also had difficulty breathing and their skin would turn to a strange shade of blue. They would die shortly after contracting the disease. This occurrence puzzled the doctors at the Tokyo military hospital because most of the soldiers were previously very healthy.

In the end, the pandemic caused the deaths of over 600,000 people in the four islands that constitute Japan. Japan had witnessed many epidemics since the Heian Era, but none had disrupted the society to the extent that the Spanish flu did. This pandemic caused the death of young people, while other epidemics seemed to spare them. The Spanish flu also spread rapidly and it did not respond to traditional remedies that tamed the other diseases. Schools were closed due to many students and members of staff being sick and unable to attend.

The country had a poor economy, which greatly affected the availability and dissemination of information. The country's newspapers such as *The Times of Japan* released information on how to curb the spread of the disease, but many people received the information too late, which cost them their lives.

People were urged to maintain a high level of hygiene and avoid unnecessary human contact so as to minimize their chances of contracting the illness. They were also advised to consume lots of green tea to boost their immune systems. Furthermore, people were asked to wear face masks while going out in public. Interestingly, the wearing of face masks remained embedded in Japanese culture. Even before the 2020 coronavirus pandemic, face masks were still part of Japanese street fashion. While the Japanese people were helpless in the face of the pandemic, they tried to avoid it at all costs.

During the pandemic, Japan was a colonial power with several states under its control. This included Korea and Taiwan, so Japan quickly spread the Spanish flu to those two colonies. In October 1918, the scourge found its way to Taiwan via Japanese soldiers. A few days after the arrival of the soldiers in Keelung Harbor, located in the northern parts of Taiwan, people started falling ill. Taiwan had a flawed public health system and this contributed significantly to the immense spread of the disease. The disease then spread to other parts of the country, and by mid-October, it had reached the city of Taipei, where 22% of the city's residents contracted the disease. The disease caused the mortality rate in the country to increase two-fold. The scourge especially caused the demise of young children under the age of 5 years. About 25,000 people died in

Taiwan due to the Spanish flu and its related complications. For the Taiwanese, it all came down to one thing: the poverty of their living conditions and the unsanitary behavior of the masses.

In Asia, each country had a unique experience with the Spanish flu pandemic. Despite causing so much pain in the Asian continent, the Spanish flu acted as an eye-opener to various communities and populations. To the native Indians, it showed them the need to be independent and in control of sensitive matters such as healthcare. To the Chinese, it proved the importance of the country's medical system. To Taiwan, it demonstrated the need for acceptable public health policy.

Until recently, the Spanish flu was the last great plague to afflict humanity in modern history. It claimed more lives than the seasonal flu. It caused more deaths than the First World War, which occurred hand in hand with it. In sum, the Spanish flu showed the world that we need to tolerate each other because more enemies could easily lead to humankind's extinction. During the Spanish flu pandemic, in their pursuit of power and influence, people forgot that managing the little they had was more important than seeking huge territories. Many countries during the time of the flu experienced the failure of their healthcare systems because most of the medical practitioners were assisting the war victims. This dearth of medical practitioners left citizens vulnerable and unable to deal with even minor medical issues.

Because of the Spanish flu, there were significant steps that were taken in understanding microorganisms and how to deal with them. In the field of medicine, there was incredible progress made in developing vaccines against the flu.

All in all, amidst the desolation caused by the flu, many lessons were learned and many important developments were made. The flu changed the world in a way that no other event could have, making the human race more conscious and careful about healthcare. It is remarkable how such an essential landmark in history has been forgotten by many. While we hope that such a scourge will never again afflict the world, the truth is that there are high chances that it will recur. Viruses are incredibly lethal microorganisms. To date, thousands of people die each year during the so-called "flu season." These people die due to flu-related complications, and this is cause for alarm, for if the typical flu virus can be that destructive, what happens when there is a new strain of flu?

As we continue to advance in the medical field, microorganisms advance in tandem by mutating. This information should always keep us working toward better healthcare, new inventions, and unending innovation.

The Spanish Flu in Oceania

Oceania is a geographical region comprising of Micronesia, Polynesia, Australasia, and Melanesia. It is made up of 14 countries, with Australia being the largest country and its city Sydney being the largest city. Oceania is distant from the Western world where the Spanish flu had its origin, but the Spanish flu still encroached and devastated this remote region. Let us try to understand how the disease reached and affected this region.

Australia is a country that may have been considered to be far remote from the places where the Spanish flu was savaging human lives. However, the country was eventually struck by the pandemic. What distinguishes Australia from other parts of the world is its relative ability to contain a virus to some extent. When the government caught wind of the pandemic that was abundant in other parts of the world, they started getting ready to protect against the virus and combat it, if necessary. There was always a point of conflict on who would conduct such endeavors, especially in a country made up of seven different states, each with its own state government. But all the states in Australia understood that preventing the disease was far more uncomplicated than dealing with its outbreak.

By July 1918, the Commonwealth Quarantine Community was convened by the Commonwealth government, requiring each state to carry out its own quarantine and isolation measures within its boundaries.

Quarantine measures were required for ships that had had contact with South Africa and New Zealand, where the Spanish flu was already affecting people. The ships were to undergo seven days' quarantine upon arrival. The first infected ships reached Australia in October 1918, and the occupants of the vessel were observed for signs of the disease and treated, if necessary, in isolation. Quarantine camps continued in operation, and by January 1919, the camps had treated over 300 cases. Unfortunately, several people died while undergoing treatment. While people were forced to wear masks while in quarantine, they were allowed limited social interactions and were under strict supervision. All these measures were done to avoid the disease's spread from one person to the other.

Furthermore, Australia had a vaccine for those who manifested signs of the killer virus. This process was vital because it strengthened the body's immunity so it could effectively fight off the virus if it attacked.

Despite all these efforts, the cunning virus was still able to move past the boundaries of quarantine camps and infiltrate the domestic population. The first case among the domestic population was cited in Melbourne. To this day, no one has been able to pinpoint the exact origin that led to a massive wildfire of virus spread in Australia. The virus continued to spread and establish itself among the resident population of Australia despite the thorough quarantine measures. This situation made some experts erroneously think that the disease was caused by a local mutating virus rather than by a more robust, more virulent virus outside the nation's borders.

Unfortunately, when the first case was detected in the state of Victoria, its government did not report immediately to the Commonwealth government. Consequently, the disease spread from Melbourne to other states. It spread to Sydney via a train. By the time the Victorian government was reporting the case (14 days later), the disease had already spread to other states. The flu had also affected a considerable number of citizens in Victoria. This incidence heightened the already existing animosity between Victoria and some other states that perceived the delay of the report as intentional and malicious.

The spread of the disease was further facilitated by soldiers who were returning from war. The isolation of the soldiers was running smoothly, but at some point, the number of soldiers overwhelmed the quarantine facilities. In one instance, a group of about 1,000 soldiers broke out of a quarantine facility in Sydney, which was unprepared for them and snake-infested. Another prominent case of troops breaking quarantine involved a soldier who was convicted to 60-days imprisonment for inciting a mutiny. When the disease had taken hold in the civilian population, land quarantine seemed to be ineffective in curbing the spread of the contagion and the disease continued to afflict the people.

In Australia, there had been strife and tension among the various states. The point of conflict was whether the country should be administrated as a whole until under a federal government or under individual state governments.

After lengthy discussions and deliberation, it was decided that each state was to enforce preventive measures against the disease. If a flu victim was noted, the Commonwealth government was to be notified immediately. But if we take another look at the first case that was reported in Melbourne, we realize that the issue was not officially reported to the Commonwealth government until 14 days had passed.

Consequently, before any restrictions could be imposed over the state of Victoria, the disease had already been transmitted to Sydney by train. This heightened the already existing animosity, possibly because the transmission of the malady to Sydney was intentional. Therefore, New South Wales closed off its borders with Victoria.

Victoria did not put in place any restrictions even after having reported the first case of the pandemic. The state of Tasmania was discontented, and for this reason, Tasmania closed its borders. Though the Spanish flu undoubtedly affected Australia's population, the mortality rate was shallow compared to other parts of the land, and most significantly, the surrounding islands.

Like other countries that had participated in the war, Australia was enduring a shortage of healthcare providers because most of them were serving at the war fronts. The remaining healthcare workers were old, disabled, and overworked. So when the pandemic set foot in the country, doctors and nurses were overwhelmed by the increasing number of cases throughout the country.

Hospitals were overwhelmed to the point of refusing to admit any more patients as they had reached full capacity. Schools that had closed down and, at times, exhibition centers and cinema halls were turned into temporary hospitals. With the scarcity of doctors and nurses, people were called upon to volunteer and help the ailing.

Tasmania was one of the islands that had put into place stringent rules in the prevention and the management of the pandemic. First of all, it completely closed off its boundaries with other Australian states or any other country. Then, it closed schools, churches, cinemas, etc. It prohibited public gatherings. As a matter of fact, church ministers would visit church followers in their homes.

Tasmania also set up enough quarantine facilities so that those who had the symptoms of the disease would be isolated and taken care of. There were repercussions for not following the rules concerning maintaining good hygiene, especially in public. The state had even gone so far as to consider punishment for those who sneezed in public. Tasmanians were urged to wear protective clothing such as face masks when going out in public.

As for Tasmania's people, they did their part. They understood that the direction the pandemic would take depended on their collective efforts, so the majority of them remained indoors. Even little children were discouraged from playing with one another. Festivities were curtailed and the general atmosphere was rather somber. Religious believers felt as though they were living during an apocalyptic period.

But all these efforts seemed to be dashed by the gods of good fortune when the state started experiencing cases of the killer disease. However, the state government, confident in their preparations, was able to manage the situation. As a result, of all the infections that occurred in Tasmania, only 171 people died. This mortality rate still remains one of the lowest rates of the Spanish flu worldwide. None of Tasmania's efforts were in vain.

New Zealand is another country in Oceania that was affected significantly by the Spanish flu. The flu is said to have been brought to the country by the prime minister, who was coming back from a war conference in Europe. Rumor had it that he pulled some strings and did not isolate himself in the quarantine facilities available to him. While that may be true, we should also consider that hundreds of soldiers were returning home from the war and these soldiers were carriers of the virus that caused the Spanish flu. Unfortunately, these soldiers did not quarantine themselves and joined their families without taking any precautions. Soon enough, there were celebrations of the war's victory all over the country, with many public gatherings and parades along the streets. All the celebrations provided excellent conditions for the Spanish flu to spread itself among the people before manifesting its telltale signs and symptoms.

About a fortnight after the return of the soldiers, people all over New Zealand started falling ill. For many, the illness began with a mild headache, then fever and chills, then muscle aches.

The signs and symptoms would escalate to vomiting, violent coughing, skin turning blue, and eventually nosebleeds and a bloody froth gushing from the nasal and oral openings. People dropped like flies. One would be healthy at breakfast, develop the flu, and pass away by dusk. The fragility of life became woefully evident. When disaster strikes, human beings tend to isolate themselves, especially if the presence of others compromises their safety. It is self-preservation in its rawest form. So the people of New Zealand retreated to their homes, and all the schools, churches, and cinema halls were closed. Shopkeepers had to shut down their businesses due to lack of clients and shortage of staff members. People tried their best to avoid the deadly contagion. but it was too late for the people to escape the Spanish flu's wrath as it had already taken root in New Zealand. The disease caused immense pain—bodily, emotionally, and mentally. Hospitals filled to the brim and temporary ones had to be set up. Doctors and nurses were overworked and laypeople had to volunteer to help in whatever way they could. Ambulances rushed up and down the country, trying to save every life they could. People asked themselves how such profound misery could follow a moment of such jubilation from winning a crucial global war?

Volunteers went from house to house, looking for the

worst cases, which were those who did not have even the strength to ask for help. At times, the volunteers would find heart-shattering situations that left them traumatized. For instance, in one of the houses, they found a husband who had bee dead for three days in his bed.

His wife was on the same bed, traumatized and unable to get up from the bed simply because she could not fathom the idea that her husband had died right next to her. The wife was sent to a mental health center while the husband was buried. Volunteers would find households with hungry and sick children whose parents had died in the same house. For this reason, people organized food carts that would feed such children and other people who could not afford food during the calamity.

The rural Maori communities of New Zealand were even more affected by the Spanish flu as compared to the native European societies of the same country. One may wonder how that could be—after all, they were all in the same region and affected by the same virus. But it is important to understand that the Maori communities may not have encountered any other influenza invasions, let alone the first wave of the Spanish flu. Therefore, they were utterly susceptible to this vicious contagion and it took a heavy toll on them. The socioeconomic conditions that this community was enduring also increased their vulnerability to the Spanish flu. With the arrival of the Europeans, the native Maori community had been pushed from their native lands. This migration meant that they had fewer grounds for hunting, gathering, and farming. In such circumstances, their diet was poor and so their immunity was weak. They also had poor and crowded residential areas. Moreover, health facilities were centralized where all the European residents lived. Therefore, the pandemic ruthlessly attacked the Maori communities and caused the demise of many Maori people, especially the young and robust.

New Zealand experienced massive death and destruction during the pandemic. So many people died that there would be vehicles that would go around homes, picking up corpses and burying them in a cemetery. This would happen not once, but twice and sometimes thrice a day. Never before had the country experienced such desolation.

Have you ever heard of Waikumite? Many people think that Waikumite was a mass graveyard for people who perished due to the Spanish flu pandemic. However, Waikumite has many individually dug graves, but since they were paupers' graves, there were no memorial stones placed on top. Furthermore, the burials were done in a hurry, so no stones were placed on the burial sites. New Zealand suffered the wrath of the pandemic at its worst. However, the people of New Zealand stood together by providing for each other, consoling each other, and trying to give hope to those who were fading into sorrow and depression. The contagion had disrupted every aspect of their life, but the New Zealanders were ready to rebuild.

The Samoan islands are also fascinating to study when it comes to the effects of the Spanish flu. Western Samoa got the pandemic from a ship from Auckland, where the Spanish flu was prevalent. On October 30th, 1918, this ship docked in Western Samoa. In a matter of days, the virus was causing extreme suffering among most of the inhabitants of Western Samoa. The disease claimed the lives of the young people who constituted the majority of the working population in the agricultural sector.

The impact on the industry was so profound that the island was famine-stricken throughout 1919. The virus incapacitated nearly 92% of Samoa's adult population and killed about a quarter of the population of Western Samoa. The whole of New Zealand, including the colony of Western Samoa, lost a total of 8,573 from its original 1,150,600 inhabitants of the country.

In contrast, American Samoa did not experience the Spanish flu. The scourge never had the opportunity to reach the island due to the island's strict maritime quarantine rules. It was essentially left unscathed. One might easily say that American Samoa was lucky. Imagine not having to experience an excess loss of life and still enjoy a relatively stable economy while remaining happy and safe. It must have been everyone's wish to have been living in American Samoa during the pandemic, had they known the extent that American Samoa was left untouched by it.

The city of Auckland in New Zealand was arguably the epicenter of the Spanish flu for Oceania (excluding Australia and American Samoa). From Auckland, the disease spread to other islands surrounding New Zealand. Take, for instance, the Fiji islands, which got the flu from *SS Talune*, a ship that had departed from Auckland with a clean bill of health. This bill of health meant that the ship had not been to a place where the Spanish flu was occurring. This status was taken to mean that the crew had not been to an area with bad miasma, which could cause them to contract the disease. Therefore, the crew posed no danger of spreading the contagion to other people.

But despite having a clean bill of health, the crew of the *SS Talune* still spread the disease to the inhabitants of the Fiji islands and other parts of Western Polynesia. This put New Zealand and other states, especially Western Samoa, at loggerheads because they thought that the former was knowingly transmitting the disease to them.

All in all, the Spanish flu wreaked terror in the affected countries of Oceania. It took with it the young and healthy people in the prime of their lives. It crippled the already ailing economies of the respective states, leaving them a ton of work to do in order to regain their former functionality.

In Oceania, the most striking aspect about the Spanish flu is the difference it had on the different countries or states, depending on how well they practiced their prevention and disease-management policies. The countries that took said measures had significantly better chances at controlling the pandemic, and, consequently, its effects. For those that did not take the disease seriously, they effectively reaped what they sowed. The Spanish flu also showed how crises bring out the humanity of people, as demonstrated in

New Zealand. In contrast, it also emphasized how catastrophes may breed animosity, hatred, and suspicion between individuals or states.

Response to the 1918 Pandemic

The human race could easily qualify as the eighth wonder of the world. Despite being the same species, we are very different from each other. Consider this fact: the human race is made up of different races, which are comprised of different communities or tribes; within these tribes are even smaller and more diverse groups made up of human beings who are variant from each other. Even identical twins, who are practically photocopies of each other, are very different from each other. This realization will help us understand why individuals, communities, and nations responded to the 1918 Spanish flu pandemic the way they did. The difference in their responses will help us understand, to some extent, how the disease affected the people.

First, let us take a look at the response of the US. Being a huge country with diverse states and communities, the US clearly demonstrates the differences in response to the 1918 pandemic and the consequences that ensued. When the first case of the pandemic was reported at Camp Funston, it was characterized as a bad flu. However, by that evening, about 100 people were suffering from the same signs as those of the first patient. This incident sparked fear in people because the disease had not yet been reported in other places. The viciousness with which the disease attacked its victims caused the residents of Kansas to be on high alert. In no time, the disease was causing immense death and destruction throughout the country. It moved from the cities to the rural areas and even to the most remote regions of the country.

For instance, in Brevig mission, a remote Alaskan village, it caused the demise of more than half the inhabitants of the village. It attacked both young and old alike, causing massive deaths, eespecially of young people. Every citizen felt the impact of this scourge.

With the shortage of medical practitioners throughout the country, Americans knew that their best chance of surviving this disease was to protect themselves. After all, they knew that prevention was better than cure. The scourge prompted Americans to improve their standards of personal and general hygiene. They also took to eating foods that were believed to ward off the disease, including lemons and oranges. In addition, they wore camphor bags around their necks to protect them from the virus. US authorities also putting into place new regulations that would reduce the spread of the virus. For instance, many schools, churches, cinema halls, and theaters were closed. Public gatherings of any type were prohibited because it was well-known that interpersonal contact was the principal agent of the disease's transmission. Lastly, quarantine measures were implemented for people who had the disease, those who were in contact with afflicted people, or those who had recently traveled.

Despite all these measures, the disease infected a multitude of people. The country was experiencing a severe shortage of medical practitioners because the majority of them were working in the war-torn areas. The few remaining medical practitioners were overworked, with some of them contracting the disease and dying.

This dire state of affairs prompted some people to step up and volunteer as nurses. The addition of volunteer nurses to the healthcare system helped ease the burden on the few doctors and nurses available. Though this response was the general response of the US as a country, let us delve into how a few individual states responded to the pandemic and how this altered the impact of the disease on these particular states.

While some states acted swiftly to combat the pandemic, others took their time in responding to it, which marked a huge difference. One of the cities that was hit especially hard by the pandemic was the city of Philadelphia. The disease reached Philadelphia via a ship from Boston, heralding the second wave of the pandemic. The atmosphere was that of pure ecstasy because the country was participating in the World War. The excitement that filled the air somehow clouded people's judgment and shielded them from reality. When the deadly ship from Boston Navy docked at Philadelphia, two members of the crew died from a flu-like disease that numerous people suspected to be the infamous Spanish flu. Philadelphia authorities, however, reassured the people, telling them that this was not reflective of the pandemic. But the following day, as if to prove a point, the flu claimed fourteen more of the crew members' lives. The public health officer, Kruger, assured the people of Philadelphia that this was not the outbreak of a disease, and if it were, they would nip the epidemic in the bud. By mid-September, the flu had well established itself in the army barracks. On September 21st, several cases of contagion were reported among the civilian population. Doctors warned that this could be the beginning of an outbreak and that the authorities should take measures of protecting the people against the contagion. However, all these pieces of advice fell on arrogant deaf ears.

The ongoing war filled the majority of the people with euphoria. By this time, the city was planning a Liberty Parade to raise funds for the war. This was a great act of patriotism and support for the government's endeavors. Doctors tried their best to convince the authorities against this public gathering, given that the disease was already among the people, but no one paid heed to this. Let us not forget that Philadelphia was and still is the largest city in Pennsylvania. It also happened to be one of the most populous cities in the country. For these reasons, holding the Liberty Parade was a terrible idea in hindsight.

Nevertheless, the parade was held and the majority of Philadelphia's citizens turned up. True to the doctors' predictions, nearly a third of people who attended the parade fell ill three days after it took place. These people presented with flu-like symptoms. By the fourth day, the hospitals were overwhelmed by the massive number of patients as they had limited facilities and few healthcare providers. By the end of the week, approximately 2,600 people had perished due to the contagion.

Curiously, this still did not wake the authorities from their deep slumber. They did not realize that the stakes were too high and the number of people that could die was too much.

In fact, there was a newspaper that wrote that the nurses were managing the situation well, whereas there were but a few qualified volunteer nurses in the city.

When the disease started causing death in droves, Philadelphia's authorities belatedly accepted that the situation was getting out of hand and strict measures had to be applied. Consequently, public gatherings were prohibited, schools and cinema halls were closed, and more actions of this kind were applied far and wide. However, the disease had already infiltrated the city and it was causing untold misery, fear, and horrifying deaths that occurred merely a few hours or days after contracting the disease. The authorities had struck the iron when it was hard and cold. The people of Philadelphia were worried because, despite the government's reassurance, death was staring them in the eye. At the peak of the pandemic, the city lost over 700 people in one day. The most affected group of people were young people who would die painful and terrible deaths. This situation was very different from what had happened during typical influenza seasons where the immune-compromised, the very young children, and the elderly were the ones who were hit the hardest.

The excessive loss of lives in Philadelphia could have been prevented if the necessary measures had been taken on time. Clearly, the lesson here is that a stitch in time saves nine. Moreover, we learn that no one is ever too safe to take precautions, especially against a disease.

In stark contrast to Philadelphia, the city of St. Louis took a different route in handling the Spanish flu situation. Long before the contagion slipped into the city, quarantine centers were installed in several places. These centers included army barracks, hospitals, and other sites. Those who were arriving in the city from other areas were mandated to be isolated until proven to be healthy. These quarantine facilities played a considerable role in protecting residents from the virus.

However, one fateful day, the virus broke out in one of the army barracks and diffused to the civilian population. Fortunately, the authorities were already prepared for this. They mobilized nurses, both qualified and voluntary nurses, and a number of doctors to attend to the sick from their homes. As tedious as this process may sound, it played a massive role in the effective control of pandemic. How so? When the Spanish flu victims stayed at their own homes, it minimized the rate at which the virus was spreading. The patients couldn't infect those that they would have encountered on their way to hospitals or other non-Spanish flu patients in the hospitals. Home visits also meant that the hospitals could effectively handle other emergencies and diseases. St. Louis also closed down schools, religious places, pools, cinema halls, markets, and any other sites for public gathering. These measures seemed terrible for business, with many business owners and investors against the idea of closing everything down. However, determined to avoid the pandemic, the city authorities took a stand and had the orders executed.

But we can all agree that this temporary shutdown was a meager price to pay for the tremendous results the city had in controlling the pandemic. In the end, St. Louis survived the plague almost unscathed.

Unlike most cities, St. Louis was able to flatten the curve and this outcome was due to several factors. The first factor was being well-prepared. The city already had a plan to prevent the infiltration of the virus. When that plan failed and the virus spread, they had even a more brilliant strategy on how to manage the pandemic and, in time, contain it. The city's people were also willing to cooperate with the authorities' restrictions. Their cooperation could have been partially inspired by the grim stories of the virus's viciousness in other states. The city's people also understood the fact that the disease was highly contagious, knowing that when one member of the family got it, that could mean the demise of the whole family in the worst-case scenario. St. Louis can surely be used as a model for the ideal response to a contagion.

In San Francisco, the Spanish flu somehow managed to slip past a well-organized quarantine system. However, the virus did not have much luck taking hold because strict regulations had been put in place, making its transmission from one person to the next incredibly difficult. Moreover, infected individuals were treated in isolation. People were to maintain high standards of hygiene, especially in public. Coughing in public was a legal reason for punishment.

Public gatherings were prohibited. When in public, people were mandated to wear gauze masks. The masks were said to be almost fully effective against the virus.

Moreover, failure to wear the gauze masks or wearing them improperly was a criminal offense. One would be charged with "disrupting the peace", which would lead to prosecution and a fine of five dollars (a lot of money in that era).

San Francisco did exceptionally well in controlling the first two waves of the Spanish flu pandemic. This may have caused people to have a false sense of complacency. On November 21st, a whistle was blown and the war against the Spanish flu was declared to be over. People threw all caution to the wind. Public gatherings were allowed once again, with schools and other institutions reopening. Everything seemed to be well until all hell broke loose in January when the third wave of the pandemic began.

Having been spared by the first two waves of the Spanish flu pandemic, the people of San Francisco, developed the misconception that gauze masks were actually effective in preventing the transmission of the virus. In truth, the masks in question were almost ineffective when it comes to curbing the spread of the virus. It was the other precautions, especially lockdowns, the shutdown of places of social amusement, and the prohibition of social gatherings that saved San Francisco's people. The people did not realize that they were making a colossal mistake until their death rate was skyrocketing. This circumstance is a classic example of what the World Health Organization (WHO) is warning people against today—celebrating too early. Experts estimate that 90% of San Francisco's deaths during the third wave of the Spanish flu could have been prevented if the people had continued with the same precautions taken during the earlier phases of the pandemic. They paid a hefty price for their complacency.

It has been said that change is inevitable, and if we don't change, the change will change us. In Spain, we can observe how rigidity in some matters may bring suffering. The Spanish flu got its name not because it originated in Spain but because Spain was the first country to speak up about it. The disease was also referred to as the "Spanish lady." As Spain was reporting on the disease, all the grotesque pain and suffering people were going through was evident. The physical, mental, and emotional distress for the victims and their loved ones was unfathomable and petrifying. But what if some of this pain could have been eliminated if a part of the society decided to be somewhat flexible?

For instance, the town of Zamora was among those that were most affected by the Spanish flu pandemic in Spain. It suffered many deaths and its people went through excruciating pain and agony. However, if the church had been more flexible in handling the situation, so many lives could have been saved. When the Spanish government was doing a crackdown on public gatherings, they closed schools, theaters, regulated markets, prohibited political meetings, and so forth. Basically, they touched on every public gathering apart from church gatherings, particularly

Mass. One may wonder why this happened. In that era, in Spain, the church had decision-making powers in the government.

Therefore, when the government tried to ban church services, the bishop said that they were interfering unnecessarily with the church's matters. As such, Holy Mass was held every day despite the ongoing pandemic. As if to add fuel to the fire, the mass was held every day and many people attended in "in search of consolation from God during these difficult times."

In Zamora, the death toll due to the Spanish flu was higher than anywhere else in Spain. Every day, there would be a burial in the town. But the people held to their belief that the pandemic was a punishment from God and that only God's mercy could deliver them. This situation shows us how superstition can lead to severe repercussions. Given that matters of faith may be sensitive, religious authorities should try to convince their followers to do what is right for them and others, especially during pandemics.

Some nations took to completely isolating themselves from the rest of the world to avoid contagion. A good example is American Samoa. The geographical location of the country naturally kept it isolated from many countries. The government effected a five-day maritime quarantine for all the boats arriving at the island. This practice literally kept the virus at bay.

Eventually, only a few people were infected, but no one

died from the disease. Tasmania imposed a full lockdown on all its borders, which managed to keep the virus out of the country for ample time.

Furthermore, even when the disease sneaked into the country, it afflicted just a few people. Moreover, the death toll of the disease in the state was among the lowest in the world. In Tasmania, only 171 people died due to the Spanish flu.

The above examples show us the different responses to the pandemic and the consequences of each response. Contrary to popular opinion, survival for the fittest was not for human beings living during the Stone Age or for wild animals. It is a continuous process that becomes more evident when catastrophes occur. Nature brings obstacles our way that we need to overcome for us to live and see another day, and eventually to perpetuate our species. This may be as simple as literally taking a breath, or as trying as surviving a pandemic. This development in almost every sector is both a blessing and a curse.

The ease of accessibility to practically every part of the globe made the spread of the 2020 coronavirus pandemic very simple. One moment, it's an epidemic in Wuhan, and the next, it's in your town. Now the virus has affected almost every citizen in the world, with only a few states and regions that haven't yet reported cases of the disease. As with the 1918 Spanish flu pandemic, the coronavirus pandemic has caused suffering throughout the world and immense destruction.

However, with improved methods of protecting ourselves from the virus, we can avoid contracting the illness. Among the many lessons to learn from the past are the also mistakes that we should never repeat.

We should exert ourselves to fight against the virus, help each other, and follow the WHO's directives. During this pandemic, nature requires us to strive to see another day, and the best way to do so is by avoiding the virus. Even when things may seem grim, let us remember that unlike 1918, we have antiviral therapy, we can develop vaccinations, and we know exactly what we are dealing with—a deadly virus. Above all, we have hope and we have each other. Though we may be separated from each other, technology connects us virtually, and we can stand in solidarity with each other because though we are apart, we are never alone.

Methods of Prevention and Treatment of the Spanish Flu

Destruction and desolation comprise an understatement of the Spanish flu's effects on the globe. With the exception of a few places, the "Spanish lady" roamed the world far and wide, and wherever she went, people could not help but tremble in fear and try their best to avoid her. The disease attacked one and all, and at the end of the day, the result was immense suffering and the demise of many individuals. Some communities had no idea of a global pandemic that was ongoing until it had already affected them. For such communities, preventing the disease from infecting them at first was difficult and most of the community members ended up dead.

A good example of such communities is the Alaskan communities in the US and several African communities. For other communities, ignorance of the gravity of the "Pale Rider" and the belief that the disease was just a misconception caused them not to take early enough precautions. This behavior cost many people their lives— for instance, in Philadelphia.

Other communities were fully aware of the gravity of the situation and they enforced measures to keep the disease at bay, thereby saving a multitude of lives. Despite these measures being enforced, if the individuals did not go to the trouble of protecting themselves, all this measures' efforts would could be in vain, Let us try to understand how various people protected themselves from the pandemic.

As they say, cleanliness is second to godliness, and do not underestimate the importance and power of cleanliness. The first line of defense against the Spanish flu pandemic was the improvement of personal hygiene. Good personal hygiene minimized the risk of contracting the disease. Even if one came in contact with the disease, good hygiene lowered the chances of being infected by it. Proper cleaning of hands, clean and well-ventilated rooms, clean clothes, and food worked remarkably well in keeping the virus at bay. During the Spanish flu pandemic, many soaps were produced, each claiming the power to kill the Spanish Flu pathogen. Disinfectants were recommended to be used in homes and in public places to deactivate the disease.

Physical distancing rules were also enforced in the course of the Spanish flu pandemic. Doctors explained that the disease could be spread from one person to the next via droplets and secretions from the mouth and nose. For this reason, the people were asked to stay away from each other. For some people, this was easy, but for some communities, this was a new challenge that required commitment. In some communities, their form of salutation is hugging, kissing, and shaking hands, and so physical distancing put an end to all that. Adapting to such a change must have been hard for them. Likewise, in other communities, meals were shared on the same plate and the pandemic required each of them to use their own plate. People had to strive to make adjustments for their own good.

People understood that the disease was a real threat, and if, they contracted it, they would have to have a robust immune system to fight against it and, hopefully, survive. To improve their immunity, people ate foods that were known to boost the immune system. These included lemons, oranges, and other citrus fruits, which were known to be effective against the typical flu. The logic behind their eating these fruits is that these fruits contain vitamin C, which is essential in fighting against disease-causing microorganisms. People also gargled warm salty water in order to get rid of the virus.

Unfortunately, as there were no known effective drugs against the virus, many people perished just a short while after contracting the disease. However, doctors recommended aspirin to alleviate the symptoms because the doctors knew no cure for this fast-acting killer disease. However, instead of curing the disease, most of the patients who used aspirin died of the Spanish flu. Most of the deaths that occurred in October 1918 are said to have been sped up by aspirin. To understand why aspirin, a highly effective drug, could have caused the highest number of deaths, we need to understand aspirin toxicity. Aspirin toxicity is caused by taking an overdose of the drug. Doctors today recommend that the maximum amount of aspirin that should be taken in a day is 4 mg. However, doctors in 1918 administered over 30 mg of aspirin in a day, and this dosage caused aspirin toxicity. Aspirin toxicity is characterized by the following signs and symptoms: hyperventilation, tinnitus, and irritation of the gastrointestinal tract. Patients may also experience nausea, vomit, have stomachaches, and bleeding.

Patients may also suffer from fevers, dizziness, and restlessness. Excess aspirin attacks the cerebral respiratory centers, which eventually causes the inhibition of the citric-acid cycle. The overall effect is that aspirin toxicity takes a heavy toll on the respiratory system, causing fluid build-up in the lungs that causes patients to suffocate.

So rather than alleviating the signs of the disease, aspirin increased its intensity, speeding the pace at which the patients approached their demise. To make matters worse, when the drug failed to work, doctors multiplied the dosage, thus increasing the drugs' harmful effects. Aspirin toxicity essentially made the disease overwhelm the patients, resulting in their deaths. As the saying goes, people perish due to lack of knowledge.

Some countries had little or no access to modern medicine. For such countries, the only resort when it came to dealing with the disease was traditional medicine. Such communities included a number of African communities, Chinese, and most Alaskan communities. Many communities in India also resorted to traditional medicine because colonialists neglected modern medical facilities, and the medical sector was not well-developed. Moreover, the majority of the Indian people did not have faith in this new modern form of medicine. Therefore, these communities had an elaborate way or ways of dealing with outbreaks and diseases like the Spanish flu. Take, for instance, China, a country with a longstanding history of medicine. Their medicine touches almost every disease or disorder that has afflicted humans throughout known history.

Moreover, the Chinese traditional medicine had a great emphasis on disease outbreaks, otherwise known as epidemics. Therefore, this community had guidelines on what to do during the Spanish flu. Furthermore, Chinese traditional medicine prescribed a mixture of some herbal medicine that proved effective against the scourge. In the end, Chinese herbal medicine was one of the few forms of medicine that worked against the scourge. Unfortunately, other forms of traditional medicine failed to work against the virus. Many people lost their lives, and all doctors and caregivers could do was watch helplessly.

When human beings cannot explain an event, many of them attribute it to the supernatural. The case was not different during 1918 pandemic. Some people believed that the disease was a punishment from God, while others believed that it was God's will that people face it. Repentance and praying was their course of action, with the hope that their pleas would be heard and that the disease would disappear as mysteriously as it had appeared.

Other people believed that they were living through the apocalypse and that the world was coming to an end. In these people's communities, science was barely advanced, and this can help us understand why the people chose this line of thought. For instance, in Zamora, a town in Spain, the church increased the number of services per day for people to attend. During these services, the people repented and prayed that God could grant them mercy and protect them from the scourge. Some went to the church in search of consolation from God during these challenging times.

This type of thinking was better than denying the fact that the world was going through a pandemic. Those who were in denial lived their lives without any precautions against the disease whatsoever. The majority of them ended up contracting the disease and learning the hard way.

In Africa, particularly in Kenya, the Spanish flu was well-documented to have hit the coastal area. This place was a very vital administrative area due to the presence of the port in Mombasa. For this reason, records on people's health were kept and assessed often to evaluate the threats that the Kenyan people could be facing. When the disease was first reported on the coast, the Kenyan population was urged to protect themselves by reducing physical contact and maintaining hygiene. Those that came into contact with the sick people were required to consult physicians and to quarantine to prevent spread from one person to the other. The sick people were looked after with great care and were recommended to consume paraffin oil three times a day. As unappealing as that may sound, paraffin oil was believed to help restore good health, physically, mentally, and spiritually. The sick were also advised to eat foods rich in starch and drink plenty of milk to restore their strength.

When the pandemic struck Nigeria, the colonial powers and local doctors collaborated and came up with ways to prevent the transmission of the disease. These ways mainly consisted of quarantine measures.

The colonial government encouraged the people to report the Spanish flu cases as they believed that with this information, they could trace, treat, and contain the disease. The government also came up with medical passes, which were documents that showed that one had not yet contracted the disease. While the passes were effective in the early phases of the pandemic, it became almost impossible to issue them when the pandemic struck many places in Nigeria. This turn of events meant that the government had to put in more effort in order to reach those who were already afflicted as well as help those who had not yet contracted the disease.

The colonial government eventually gave police officers permission to access private homes in search of infected people and take them to healthcare centers. The mandate may have been suggested in good faith, but many people ended up being mishandled and ill-treated by the officers. The searches were unpredictable and, therefore, inconvenient for the people. This method was mostly used in Lagos, where it bred mistrust and consequent hostility between the civilians and the authorities. For this reason, many inhabitants fled the city in search of a better place. As they were moving, some of them carried the virus with them, consequently and unknowingly spreading it to other people. Others went to seek solace in virus-infected areas and caught the Spanish flu in the process. All in all, this method did more harm than good. Due to the lack of trust, the method was not able to yield good results. On the contrary, it propagated the spread of the disease.

The pandemic was new to everyone around the globe and the responses to it was different. Some of the methods worked while others flopped. Even the methods that worked on some people failed terribly in others. It was basically a matter of trial and error.

At the same time, there were new and innovative methods that were truly therapeutic. An example of such methods was the use of open-air hospitals in Britain. Realizing that a great deal of patients died in the typical hospitals, some doctors suggested that the patients suffering from respiratory diseases should be taken outside and be treated in open-air hospitals. One might wonder what advantages these hospitals would have. It was an outlandish idea, but he open-air hospitals had several advantages. First, there was excellent airflow outside. Therefore, the diseases were not transmitted from one patient to another, assuming that the patients were admitted for different reasons.

Moreover, doctors were protected from contracting the various diseases that they were treating. This form of treatment also helped the patients to avoid nosocomial infections. Nosocomial infections are infections one catches from a hospital that they didn't have while being admitted to the hospital. All in all, the treatment method was found to have many advantages to the patients. Doctors reported that the patients improved physically and mentally. This new method of treatment offered great hope to sick people and their families.

In South Africa, the disease afflicted all, regardless of gender, race, and class. The disease was spreading like wildfire and the health facilities were overwhelmed. As a result, the government decided to decentralize the health system. The government divided the country into districts in an attempt to improve healthcare. This decision helped a great deal because many more people could access the available medical facilities. Though this step infuriated the apartheid supporters, at the end of the day, it helped everyone no matter their race. The disease was ravaging the population, particularly Black people who were living in deplorable conditions. In cities, Black people were the primary occupants of the townships. Crowded, unsanitary, and underdeveloped, townships provided the perfect grounds for the transmission of the disease from one person to the next. The poor people living in them suffered the most because, despite that the health centers were decentralized, the townships were lucky if they had access to any health center. The township's people were living in abject poverty. They could barely afford meals and getting healthcare services was almost impossible for them. About 300,000 South Africans died due to the Spanish flu pandemic, making South Africa among the top five countries affected by the Spanish flu.

In almost all African nations, healthcare facilities were inadequate and without the necessary facilities. When the disease struck most of the African countries, hospitals were easily overwhelmed by the massive influx of patients. The available staff was also undertrained, and this lack of training also made it very difficult to help the victims of the 1918 scourge.

Many people died due to lack of professional care. Also, due to the scarcity of hospitals, makeshift hospitals were put up in classrooms, churches, chief's camps, and other areas. Many people were treated at such places in the hope that they would resume their normal lives. But sadly, most of these victims, especially the young men and women in their prime, lost their lives. Some African people sought out herbal medicine, hoping that it would cure the disease. Despite all these efforts, the scourge trampled over Africa, killing many and leaving behind orphaned children, hopeless people, and a weak economy.

Coastal towns in most parts of the world were aware that they were a potential entry point for the disease. Therefore, the authorities put in place stringent lockdowns at the harbors and also quarantines for ships that were bringing in goods. The ports did a reasonably good job when it came to monitoring the incoming ships. However, if and when the Spanish flu infiltrated the ports, most people responded by fleeing the ports to the inland. The same happened in cities; if the disease were detected, people would flee to the countryside. This trend promoted the rapid spread of the disease. Ultimately, the disease established itself in almost every part of the globe.

In every approach used in the various parts of the world, there were critics of it. This is par for the course because, as human beings, we have diversity in the way we see and do everything. One of the measures that faced massive opposition was the mandated wearing of masks in public.

Even during the 2020 global pandemic of coronavirus, this measure has faced significant opposition throughout the world. In 1918, in San Francisco, the anti-maskers protested throughout the city, demanding that mask-wearing should be made optional. Eventually, mask-wearing was made optional by the authorities. But this newfound "freedom" had a dark side—in January 1919, San Francisco lost thousands of people to the third wave of the Spanish flu pandemic. This massive loss could have been reduced by 90% if the people had persisted in wearing masks for somewhat longer. Before opposing any measure against disease management in our modern world, we should consider the advantages and repercussions. With our scientific advancements, we can easily come to a good conclusion after considering the research.

In an age where viewing viruses in a microscope was not yet possible, management of the Spanish flu was quite a task. People experienced a major setback in considering that they thought that the disease was bacterial. There was no antiviral medication back then. Thus, people had to endure the excruciating damage caused by the virus. Treating the symptoms of the disease was akin to trying to extinguish smoke while a fire was still ablaze. The symptoms could disappear for a while before reappearing, stronger and more persistent. With no vaccine in place, the disease was a threat to human life.

All the efforts that each person took in the prevention and the treatment of this strange malady should be appreciated.

People of this time suffered from the lack of knowledge—in fact, many of them perished, and this was costly. Some of the methods that were used propagated the disease further as opposed to people's expectations. The disease, however, prompted the people in the field of medicine to do more research concerning the disease. It continued to cause a shudder when people recalled it. Even after a decade passed, scientists were still digging into it and they finally discovered its causative agent, the influenza virus. From this point, it was just a matter of building on this information until we obtained full information about this scourge.

As a disease that occurred in fairly recent history, the Spanish flu enlightens us on possible methods that could be used to conquer another pandemic. It also shows us the effective methods and those that are ineffectual. This does not mean that we will not make mistakes in this ongoing coronavirus pandemic or in a future pandemic. However, if we make them, it will be due to arrogance other than ignorance. We also need to know that the people back then did their best with what they had. With a vast sea of resources and a million possibilities, we are even more capable of dealing with the 2020 coronavirus pandemic or any other pandemic that may come our way. All we need to do is stay calm, fight the battle, and learn the lessons.

The Effects of the Spanish Flu

The 1918 Spanish flu pandemic was a monstrous catastrophe. It had casualties throughout the world. The chaos it caused was both quiet and lethal. It claimed more lives than a couple of significant wars combined. In the span of two years, it had already surpassed the damage that the Black Death did in over one decade. The Spanish flu had an immense impact on all areas of life and only the lucky few did not feel the terror caused by the scourge.

The disease caused the deterioration of the health of all individuals; young or old, and from every race, creed, and religion. It also had a significant impact on the mental health of individuals. Remember that the pandemic occurred simultaneously as the First World War, so people were already worried about losing their lives, and here was another life-threatening issue. The two years of the pandemic were marked by utter restlessness and tension among the masses. Everyone was living in fear of contracting the disease, and those who were already suffering from it were anxious that they would perish. The person next to you could transmit the disease to you, so people became suspicious of each other. What an exhausting period to live in! Quite naturally, the disease caused the decline of mental, physical, and spiritual health.

However, the disease prompted numerous advancements in the field of medicine. It sped up the discovery of an effective vaccine against influenza. Moreover, it prompted the realization of aspirin toxicity as a life-threatening issue.

People also learned about infectious disease management post-Spanish flu, with these lessons being applied in the management of diseases such as Ebola and the swine flu. The Spanish flu also shed light on the need to focus on restoring of holistic health, not only physical health but also emotional, mental, and spiritual health. The pandemic directly impacted the health sector and these were just some of its effects.

The Spanish flu had a resounding effect on the social lives of people. Society at large changed tremendously from what it was before the pandemic occurred. To start with the realm of social interactions, forms of salutation were greatly affected. Social-distancing rules were in place, and they stipulated against some forms of salutations such as hugging and kissing. We may assume that this change did not affect the people's mentality, but it certainly did. It affected the way people related to each other.

Places of worship and other areas of social interaction were closed. This, coupled with the prohibition of public gatherings, greatly affected the way people related to and interacted with each other. For some people, these were the places they met and strengthened the bonds of their relationship. The closure of these places meant that they would no longer meet, which killed familiarity and led to many of these relationships not surviving the pandemic. Meeting in places of worship brought people together and brought harmony among them. People also felt a sense of comfort when in communion with the supernatural.

The pandemic took away this part of their lives, leaving people to pray in their homes, by themselves or with their families. Some people became more deeply rooted in their faith, whereas lost their faith, seeing that no form of intervention seemed to work against the disease.

For some communities, the pandemic played a significant role in uniting them to fight against the pandemic. In New Zealand, people were united more than ever before in light of combatting the Spanish flu. They understood that while united, they could easily fight the disease. They helped sick people in hospitals and at home. People provide food for those who were not in a position to earn their daily bread, including orphaned children and extremely sick adults. They also helped to respectfully dispose of the bodies of the deceased. By the end of the pandemic, New Zealand's community members had improved their relationships with each other by showing more compassion and consideration.

Self-preservation is one of the most basic human instincts. It compels us to do whatever we can in order to be alive, even if sometimes means tearing ourselves apart from what and whom we know. This was the case in some parts of the US, where people were afraid to contact other people, especially the families of those afflicted by the Spanish flu. In some homes, entire families would die, but the neighbors would be too afraid to go and bury the bodies. In other places, parents would leave behind children, hungry and crying, but no one would bother to go and look after them.

The people were too afraid of the scourge to risk their lives to help others. In such cases, only humanitarian organizations intervened and looked out for the unfortunate. This circumstance taught people that they had to be self-sufficient and that depending on others would only disappoint them. It also bred mistrust among survivors because they knew that they could not count on each other.

When the Spanish flu pandemic struck, inoculation became one of the ways that people prevented the flu from spreading. As time went by, the method became highly appreciated, especially by people of the upper class. In Australia, it was even deemed fashionable. People who had undergone this process, particularly socialites, showed off their arms for people to see that they had experienced the process. The Spanish flu also influenced fashion. This was especially true in Japan, where people continued to wear masks long after the pandemic was gone. Masks became part and parcel of Japanese street fashion.

The Spanish flu affected the lives of children in a major way. These children had played with each other all their short lives, but now they had to stay indoors. The majority of them were discouraged from coming into contact with each other to avoid contracting the disease. That was not all; in some families, children lost their parents to the pestilence. This tragedy necessitated that the children take up the roles of the parents and provide for the family. Most children had a hard time to process and adapt to the changes that occurred due to the Spanish flu pandemic.

Schools were also closed, meaning that the children's social life was abruptly disrupted. They would no longer meet their schoolmates. Schools played a significant role in the educational and character development of children, as they do today. So when these children stayed at home, some of them did not acquire character development, especially in terms of expressing themselves.

The Spanish flu almost shattered an overall sense of community, something that people had known for ages. Some communities that were living in larger communes had to disassemble them and live as individual families. This change robbed them of their sense of belonging and the enriching company of each other. To make matters worse, when people were infected, they were isolated from their families. The only people that graced them with their presence were the caregivers who came by only a few times a day. Some of these people died in utter anxiety, desolation, and hopelessness. On the contrary, this separation helped other people to find themselves and grow as individuals.

The Spanish flu decimated life expectancy. Catching the Spanish flu was seen as being already dead, as the disease rarely spared a soul. The young men and women were those who were mostly affected by this scourge. In the US, it reduced life expectancy by a dozen years. The Spanish flu shattered society's idea of the ideal scene of death. In many societies, even today, the ideal way to part with the world is when one is grey and old, surrounded by family, or while serving the country at times of war—but the pandemic spat on this part of human dignity.

Many victims of the Spanish Flu were young people with their whole lives in front of them versus the elderly.

Moreover, the victims, more often than not, died deaths full of misery and desolation in isolated hospital wards. They left behind families in great anxiety and misery—what a cruel way to leave the world.

The Spanish flu influenced culture and culture influenced the disease. Due to this life-threatening disease, people had to give up some aspects of their lives, at least for a short time. These aspects included visiting places of worship. Those who did not change this part of their lives ended up being infected by the disease. It was a matter of changing the ways of their lives or paying the price that comes with rigidity, and those who chose the latter ended up dead.

The Spanish flu also had a huge impact on the politics of the world. The fact that it came about during a global war meant that it could easily make or break a nation's position in world politics. The war directly altered the cause of the First World War. It affected the activity of soldiers on either side of the war because the soldiers could not fight while sick. In a way, it mollified the effects that the first World War could have had because it attacked both sides of the war, leaving behind sick soldiers who were struggling to survive.

In Nigeria, it bred hostility between the locals and the colonial government due to the colonial government's stringent measures against the people.

It gave Nigerian natives the urge to be in control of their own country again.

In India, the Spanish flu pandemic brought to light the selfishness of the colonial government. The government blamed Indian natives for the disease. Furthermore, the colonialists had failed to develop the health sector and the malady took a heavy toll on the Indian population. The arrogance with which the colonial government treated the Indians during this pandemic, coupled with their oppression, made the Indians work harder at the struggle for their independence. Leaders such as Mahatma Gandhi worked to keep this fire burning. Though the process took quite some time, India finally got its freedom, largely thanks to the experience they endured during the pandemic. For most nations under colonial rule, the Spanish flu worked as an equalizer of all because it afflicted all. The oppressor and the oppressed were all bearing the yoke of the scourge. Bearing this fact in mind, the native Indians realized that the colonialists were people like them who could be easily conquered. They came to the realization that the colonialists had no power whatsoever over them.

The flu affected all people equally. For this reason, some people called it the "democratic disease." It could infect kings and rulers and commoners alike. No one seemed to crack the code on how to bring this monstrosity down. It brought out the vulnerability of human beings, no matter who they were.

This invisible enemy reminded the people that before having designations of class, gender, color, creed, or religion, they were first and foremost human beings. It reminded them to look out for each other and that each one of them deserved respect.

The disease may have disrupted the existing forms of government in some areas of the world. For instance, in Australia, when the Australian states closed their borders, the federal government was ignored for some time during the pandemic. Each of the state governments was operating as its own unit. Prevention, management, and treatment of the cases of the disease were done within the states. Some states were highly effective in their management, while others flopped. Comparing the management of the disease in Tasmania and Victoria clearly demonstrates that fact. The Spanish flu pandemic highlighted that the states could run smoothly on their own, but they also needed each other, especially in an economic sense.

As in India, many other colonialists let the scourge devastate the native people. These colonial powers did next to nothing to prevent the entry and spread of this pestilence. The disease took a hefty number of lives. In Philippines, for example, the American colonial government imposed no protective measures against the Spanish flu and the island lost close to 80,000 natives. In this way, the colonialists were able to control the people to impose their political agenda.

The Spanish flu provided a platform the people could use to exercise their rights. This platform would arise when people were in opposition to the methods used to curb the disease. In San Francisco, in 1918, anti-maskers demanded that mask-wearing should be made optional. People were granted this demand because the state is a democratic one, and indeed, the majority has their way. Even though the effects of the revocation of the law were harmful, this move showed the people of San Francisco that they could demand change in this way.

Studying the impact of the Spanish flu on the economy is more difficult because there is little or no documentation of this type of impact. However, considering that the disease mostly caused the demise of the young and robust, the crippling of the economy was evident. It could be witnessed and felt everywhere. On a firsthand basis, some families lost their sole breadwinners, and this lowered their standard of living. Scarcity of food was reported almost everywhere around the globe. For instance, in India, a severe famine attacked the people in 1919. The famine meant that people were malnourished and, consequently, immuno-compromised, and the disease hit them especially hard. In Kenya, settlers and natives alike suffered food shortages. The people who were supposed to work the farms were sick, which led to a terrible food shortage. Malnourished and weak, people fell prey to the Spanish flu and many of the victims eventually succumbed to the disease. The flu took away their quality of life and made it all about striving to see another day.

In the US, shopkeepers and other businesspeople were against the lockdown of the country. This was not because they did not understand the gravity of the situation, but their businesses suffered immensely because of the reduced number of customers that they were getting on a daily basis. This decline meant that there was little cash flow and some goods went bad. The grocery-store business in many US states declined by about a third. In department stores, they made less than half of the returns that they made before the pandemic began. It was a time of great crisis, especially for small and medium enterprises.

Contrary to expectation, the overall effect of the 1918 pandemic on the economy was somewhat mild. This was because the country had already undergone a decline earlier and the pandemic's effects were just a continuation of the same trend. Moreover, some companies were making huge profits due to the pandemic. These included fumigation companies, mask manufacturers, and detergent companies that provided tools to eliminate the virus. Moreover, due to the increasing number of patients in hospitals, companies such as pharmaceutical companies, mattresses and bedding companies, and other such manufacturers made good money that year. The profits made by these companies filled the void that was left by other businesses.

In countries such as South Africa, the economic impact was particularly devastating. As a country whose economy relies on mining and agriculture, the country suffered.

The pandemic took a hefty toll on the people at the prime of their lives—people who provided labor and expertise in their various fields. During the pandemic, 33% of the workers would be absent each day. This absence meant that there would be less production on that day, which translated to huge losses for the country. In the mines, the stuffy conditions of the tunnels facilitated the spread of the disease. Many miners came down with the flu. The decline in the workforce directly affected the amount of the minerals mined and, eventually, the returns from that work.

The pandemic did not spare industries in Britain. Some workers could not report to work because of the disease. As if this was not enough disruption, other workers would suddenly fall ill and die after a short while due to the virus. This turn of events affected the productivity at industries because even those who were still healthy were too traumatized to work effectively. Many industries shut down due to this attitude. It is worth remembering that the availability of raw materials was minimal during this time, and some industries shut down because they had nothing to work on. When such effects befall the economy of a country, the GDP falls. Many more people live below the poverty line. Basic needs become hard to acquire, and more often than not, the rate of crime skyrockets. Such an increase in crime rates was reported in many parts of the world.

The Spanish flu affected the economy and the economy affected the Spanish flu. As the Spanish flu was causing the economy to decline, the struggle to maintain the economy promoted the spread of the disease. For instance, in the US, some sectors of production continued to operate so as to keep up with the increased demand for the products. In these industries, social-distancing rules were not put into consideration and the disease spread easily in factories and to anyone who interacted with the factory workers. Eventually, the disease gripped many of the workers. Owing to this effect, various mines and industries were on the verge of a lockdown when the pandemic was coming to an end.

In Australia, the state of Tasmania experienced a sharp economic decline due to its complete lockdown. The imposing of a lockdown meant that the state could not participate in any forms of trade with other Australian states or other parts of the world. The situation was the same in many other countries. When the lockdown measures were stringent, cases of the disease were few and manageable. A declining economy was definitely a small price to pay to protect the people.

The monstrosity that was the Spanish flu had a great impact on the lives of people. Although the effects were watered down by the infamous first World War, the impacts of the pandemic can be observed in our society, particularly in the medical field. Though it is referred to as the forgotten pandemic, we must keep its memory alive, learn from it, and, above all, avoid making the same mistakes done by our predecessors.

Misconceptions about the 1918 Flu Pandemic

The Spanish flu pandemic was a phenomenon that shook the earth to its core. It has been called the greatest pandemic in modern history. Being so infamous for the destruction it caused, there has been a lot of information in the media concerning the disease. Some of it is true, while a big chunk of this information is just a product of a wild imagination or fear.

The first misconception about the disease actually springs from the name of the pandemic. Many people liken coronavirus with the slur the "Wuhan Virus" or the "Chinese Virus." Similarly, the Spanish flu did not originate from Spain, but from either Kansas or northern China. The disease was associated with Spain because the Spanish media was not censored. Rather, the country openly spoke out about the hefty toll the disease was taking on its population. They described it as a strange flu-like malady that attacked many people in Madrid. They described how it spread from cities to rural areas and even to the remotest parts of Spain. Soon enough, the disease afflicted the king and several officials of the government. Since Spain was the only one that reported these cases, it seemed to be contained to that country, but in reality, other countries were equally suffering. They just chose not to speak about it. So that's our first myth debunked: the 1918 pandemic did NOT originate from Spain.

Is the 2020 global pandemic of coronavirus going to have a second wave? Even before you finish typing it, Google will complete this question for you because people have already Googled it all over the world. This is due to fear that the disease may follow the trend set by the infamous Spanish flu. It is true that the 1918 pandemic occurred in three distinct waves. The main misconception concerning the 1918 pandemic occurrence is that the first wave was the most vicious and caused more damage than any other wave. In truth, the first wave of the Spanish flu was a mild one. It caused the same symptoms of the typical seasonal flu such as coughing, headache, fever, and a runny nose. These symptoms were nothing out of the ordinary, and in many parts of the world, it was mistaken for a typical flu outbreak.

The second wave of the Spanish flu was the deadliest phase that characterized the virulence of Spanish flu. It attacked with the viciousness of a snake and killed with the speed of lightning. This phase occurred between October 1918 and December 1918. It accounted for more than half of all the deaths that occurred due to the Spanish flu. As for the signs and symptoms, we could say that this phase brought out the Spanish flu's dramatic side. It was characterized by signs of the typical flu in a larger magnitude and a firmer grip on the victim's body.

Moreover, the disease manifested cyanosis, or the condition of a lack of oxygen throughout the body, making the skin turn blue. The disease could kill in just a matter of hours after one contracted it.

This pace left no room for intervention. In its second phase, the Spanish flu showed no mercy on its victims – it particularly targeted those who were in the prime of their lives with a long life ahead of them and the pillars of their society. Their deaths left the world in a desolate state, especially economically, as these young people had been the main drivers of the economy.

The 1918 pandemic was lethal and it killed mercilessly. There was neither a cure nor a vaccine for Spanish flu, which probably meant that no form of remedy was effective against the disease, right? Wrong. Today, many people think that home-care remedies were ineffective against the disease, as during this period, hospitals were a luxury mainly for the rich and affluent. The available hospitals were also overcrowded and with fewer facilities, making them a propagator of the disease.

One of the primary forms of treatment that people resorted to was traditional medicine. This form of medicine involved a great deal of home-care remedies and general hygiene. For most patients, it worked to alleviate the signs and symptoms. However, we should remember that, unlike the typical flu, whose signs and symptoms can be suppressed by essential home remedies until the flu subsides, the Spanish flu was much stronger. Though it's true that home-care remedies alleviated some signs and symptoms, they did nothing to the stronger and more infectious virus, and this is the main reason why it did not get any recognizable results. The symptoms would subside for a short time, then come back much stronger.

Moreover, home-care remedies were often coupled with mega-doses of aspirin, which eventually caused aspirin toxicity that did far more harm than good. Aspirin toxicity worsened the symptoms of the disease, increasing the likelihood of death.

However, in China, traditional Chinese medicine seemingly worked like magic. In this country, they registered a 97% recovery rate of Spanish flu cases at the peak of the pandemic. This trend shows us clearly that home-based care and remedies sometimes worked for people with the Spanish flu.

Having heard the effects of the 1918 pandemic, we may be tempted to think that a "super virus" caused the disease. However, this is not the case. The disease was actually caused by a more virulent strain of the influenza virus. Namely, it is the type A influenza virus, subtype H1N1. The virus was more virulent because it was a new strain that came forth after mutating. Its mutating gave it better adaptation in order to enter human cells.

Moreover, the virus could evade the body's immune system, thereby weakening the body. Another factor that could have increased the virus's impact on the body was the lack of previous exposure to the disease. A theory was developed stating that the disease affected mostly young people because they did not experience the Russian flu. The Russian flu was a pandemic that occurred in the late 1800s.

Exposure to this pandemic is thought to have given the elderly a vantage point when combatting the Spanish flu, particularly the second wave of the flu. Still, from this perspective, we observe that the pestilence took a severe toll on the native communities. These people had no previous exposure to influenza. Therefore, the disease weakened, destroyed, and devastated their bodies. All in all, let us understand that the disease was just a typical virus that mutated, thus having the capacity to overwhelm the body quickly.

As we know by now, the pandemic coincided with the First World War. For this reason, many people assume that the disease changed the course of the war. This information may seem real because the disease certainly afflicted soldiers; in fact, soldiers carried it from Kansas to Europe. The disease weakened soldiers and incapacitated them so that they could no longer fight, raising an issue that could have affected the war in a huge way. However, the soldiers were under pressure that this was a global war, and therefore they strived to fight in the best way they could. Moreover, the disease attacked and weakened both sides of the war, thereby creating a zero net effect. Though the disease impacted the war, the impact was not significant enough to change the course of the war.

It is normal to hear that the Spanish flu killed most of the people who were infected. Frightening to hear, right? The truth of the matter is that this pandemic infected about a third of the world's population.

This fraction translates to about 500 million people, and this is a huge number. Of all the infected persons, about 50-100 million people died. This number may sound massive, but in a real sense, only 20% of all the infected people died. This means that the larger number of the pandemic's victims actually came out alive. In fact, in some places such as China, traditional medicine worked effectively against the disease and there was almost 100% recovery from the Spanish Flu. Therefore, though the pandemic was undoubtedly devastating, several people survived and lived to tell the story of escaping from the jaws of death. The communities that suffered the most deaths from the pandemic were the native communities. Due to their lack of previous exposure to influenza, the disease dealt them a major blow. Among the Native American communities, entire villages were virtually wiped out by the virus. For instance, Brevig Mission in Alaska lost 72 of its residents within five days, leaving behind only eight teenagers and children as survivors. Therefore, we can say that the disease had a low mortality rate except for places that had not yet experienced any influenza outbreaks.

There is a misconception that states that vaccination is what brought the 1918 Spanish flu pandemic to an end. 1918 may sound just like a short while ago, but the truth is that that was a completely different era from today. There were just a few advancements in the field of science and medicine. Though Edward Jenner had already discovered and used vaccination, the truth of the matter is that the

Spanish flu had no vaccine. Moreover, there was no cure for the disease.

There were no antivirals. The only thing that was somewhat helpful at that time was aspirin, which alleviated the symptoms of the disease. However, doctors made the mistake of prescribing it in excess, which led it to cause aspirin toxicity. Aspirin toxicity damaged the respiratory system that was already compromised by the disease, which advanced the symptoms of the disease and frequently led to the patient's death. People also consumed some foods that would boost their immune systems. These included oranges and lemons, which have been used since time immemorial to prevent and relieve the common cold. During the Spanish flu, people used it in the hope that it would work the same way. Unfortunately, the disease managed to slip into people's bodies and cause immense havoc. Therefore, without any working remedies against the disease, patients resorted to home care. Otherwise, this was the case of "may the best immune system win." It was natural selection at its best. In sum, vaccination did not eliminate the virus from the face of the earth. In fact, the disease just died out and disappeared as mysteriously as it had appeared.

Some people are wrongly informed that no one knows the virus that caused the infamous Spanish flu pandemic. However, the virus is well-known: it is the influenza virus Type A, subtype H1N1. In 1933, the influenza virus type A was discovered. In 1951, John Hultin, a medical student, attempted to isolate the virus that caused the Spanish flu from a victim's body without success. In 1972, he traveled to Brevig's mission, an Alaskan village that was one of the places that was most hit by the pandemic. At this time, he was a retired pathologist.

With the permission of the village authorities, he unearthed the frozen bodies of several victims of the Spanish flu. Eventually, he isolated the virus that had wreaked chaos on the earth—influenza type A virus.

By 2005, the virus had been genetically sequenced and there was quite literally a full picture of the virus. Monkeys were infected with the virus, they went down with the flu and eventually died. After studying the monkey's organs, it was apparent that they died for the same reason that so many young people died in 1918—cytokine expulsion. Therefore, the virus that caused the pandemic has been studied and scientists have a full understanding of it.

Many of us now tend to compare the Spanish flu with the 2020 coronavirus pandemic. This comparison may give us the false assumption that the Spanish flu dominated the news in that era. However, we should understand that the pandemic occurred alongside with World War I when the media was censored in most countries and they focused mainly on the war. This media censorship was meant to make the people understand the gravity of the war. In the US, this mentality was promoted to mobilize the people to campaign and raise funds for the war. In Britain, people had been prohibited from making utterances that would "kill the spirit of war." Announcements concerning the scourge could only make the people live in fear, which was contrary to such spirit. Yet, it's worth emphasizing that people could see how the disease was ravaging them even though the media was barred from talking about it.

This behavior made people lose their faith in the government to some extent. It was only in Spain where the media could speak freely about the disease. They even notified their neighbors on the pestilence that was affecting people. Therefore, unlike today, people rarely heard about the disease from the news. Nevertheless, the media was not needed so much on this one. People actually suffered from the disease and had firsthand experience with it. Hearing it over the news made no difference.

The last misconception is based on probability and is as follows: the world is probably no better prepared for another pandemic than it was in 1918. This misconception compares the modern world with a world that has no idea that its pandemic was caused by a virus, a world with no antivirals and no vaccines, and a world with shortage of doctors to treat the flu victims. It puts the modern world alongside with a world that was still at the infancy of medicine, a world where more funds were used on war than on medical research. All in all, our world is better equipped to deal with a pandemic today than back in 1918. Today, it is easy to isolate and identify causative agents of disease. The technology in the world today is incomparable to the microscopes that could not show a virus in 1918. To be clear, I am not belittling the world of then—I want to help us understand that the world we are living in today is well-equipped to handle a pandemic.

Today, doctors understand how diseases are transmitted and what should be done to prevent the disease's massive spread. People need to stay calm and remember that we've got a handle on the pandemic sweeping over us today.

The above misconceptions are just a few misconceptions about the Spanish flu. In any case, when we get information that seems suspicious, especially about the ongoing pandemic, it is wise to carry out research and verify it. In today's world, research is only a click away or a flip-of a-page away, and this should encourage us to know as much as we can about things that matter to us. Remember, knowledge is power. The lack of knowledge is weakness and having false or little knowledge is destructive. Let us be enlightened and debunk these myths.

Conclusion

This book has expounded on the 1918 pandemic, touching on how it affected the world economically, socially, and politically. This study of the 1918 pandemic sheds light on how the ongoing coronavirus pandemic may affect the modern world. In a nutshell, here are the main areas of concern with the 1918 pandemic.

This pandemic was caused by the influenza virus. Namely, type A, subtype H1N1. The type A influenza virus is responsible for all the influenza pandemics that have scourged the earth. These viruses can mutate and form new strains that are more lethal than the seasonal flu.

We have learned that the Spanish flu, also known as the "Spanish Lady", did not originate from Spain. Its name derives from the fact that the media in Spain spoke out about it at a time that no other country did. The disease affected almost every part of the world, disrupting people's way of life. This disease occurred in three phases, known as waves, which were distinct from each other. Within two years, the disease claimed up to 100 million lives. This number represents 5% of the world's population. Overall, the disease infected a third of the world's population, translating to about 500 million people. Therefore, it caused immense suffering and agony to many people all over the world.

The Spanish flu attacked one and all. It attacked all the continents stretching to the most remote areas. It was particularly deadly on the communities that had not had previous exposure to influenza.

The pandemic caused a massive decline in the health of the victims. The victims became frail and thin and could not interact with others. It affected the relationships of individuals to one another. The more interaction that one had with others, the higher their chances of getting the disease. This situation made many people chose solitude for the sake of self-preservation. It changed the way people viewed religion. While some found consolation and hope in religion, others found it absurd and unhelpful during these challenging times. For most people, the world turned upside-down.

The so-called forgotten pandemic almost brought the world to a standstill. Countries locked down their boundaries. There was no flow of goods or people in or out of countries. Economies came crashing down, and people's livelihood and quality of life came down with it. The Spanish flu was a tremendously great tragedy. Everything was closed down—cinemas, schools, churches, and even businesses. The disease was really hard on the economy. It did not make matters better, considering that the First World War had done its fair share of damage to the economy.

Politically speaking, the disease helped some people find their voice in speaking up against their oppressors. The disease showed them that all human beings are equal, regardless of their profession, race, or religion. It got the nickname "the democratic disease" because it attacked one and all; the leader and the follower, ruler, and civilian; the oppressor and the oppressed.

It gave people under the yoke of colonialism a reason to fight for their independence. When it comes to politics, we could say that it did more good than harm and could be seen as a silver lining.

In short, this catastrophe touched every part of life except for the few people who were left unscathed. The most profound impact of this disease is felt in the field of medicine. The disease left behind countless lessons on how to handle infectious diseases. Specifically, it emphasized the application of strict and effective quarantine to curb the spread of infectious disease. It gave doctors and researchers a newfound zeal to devise vaccines to prevent diseases. It brought to light the importance of traditional medicine as an alternative to modern medicine.

In our more advanced world than the world of 1918, we know that a pandemic would spread faster than the 1918 pandemic given that the world is a global village. Fast means of transport can take us wherever we want in just a matter of hours, facilitating the equally quick spread of disease. Parcels can also act as a medium of transmission of pandemics, something we have already witnessed in the ongoing coronavirus pandemic. However, we do not need to panic because, unlike the Spanish flu, we are up to date with all aspects of the disease's progress. Moreover, we can identify and genetically sequence the causative agent in a short time. Having understood the causative agent, treating the disease becomes more manageable because we familiarize ourselves with it. The development of a vaccine is already underway.

Fortunately, the vaccine should be out soon as we have very knowledgeable and capable scientists.

However, it's still true that prevention is better than cure. We have to strive to evade diseases because they remain a threat to our lives. We should continue to protect ourselves and our loved ones. Even though social-distancing rules are in place, we should look out for and keep in touch with each other. We should show love and kindness to each other because living through a global pandemic is a real struggle. Keeping in mind that health comprises mental, physical, and spiritual well-being, we should take care of all these aspects.

It's a stressful time to live in, but remember that you can take that walk, listen to that song that you love, watch that movie, call that friend, and do what you feel like at home. During this time, we may feel out of touch with the world, but now is the time to declutter your life. Kill that bad habit and replace it with a more helpful one. Detoxify your body, mind, and spirit. Lose those false friends, revoke those negative thoughts, and silence that toxic voice inside of you. There are some days you will wake up and all you can do is survive. And that's OK, as we are in the middle of a pandemic, and living through the day is enough work already.

In short, keep fit, mentally, physically, and spiritually. When this is over and done, may you emerge having matured and glowing. Let us be the first generation to come out of pandemic stronger and better people.

I hope you enjoyed this book! If you like, leave a positive review with your impressions on the Amazon page. I would be really grateful! Check my other books in the Author Page on Amazon, you will find them very interesting! See you at the next reading!

For any kind of request, clarification or advice, feel completely free to contact me at the following email address: davidanversa.author@gmail.com
Thank you very much
David Anversa

Made in United States
Troutdale, OR
12/06/2023